Off the Grid With
DIABETES

What To Do If You Have Diabetes &
All Hell Breaks Loose

By Sam Adams

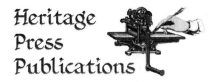

Heritage
Press
Publications

Published by:
Heritage Press Publications, LLC
PO Box 561
Collinsville, MS 39325

ISBN-13: 978-1-937660-16-1

ISBN-10: 1937660168

Table of Contents

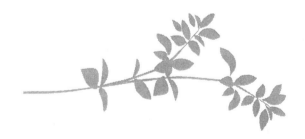

Off the Grid with Diabetes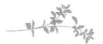

Introduction

In 2005, I learned that a global epidemic that was claiming hundreds of thousands of new victims each month had its grip on my life. My physician, a soft-spoken internist with a soothing bedside manner, delivered the news firmly but gently: I was a diabetic. My blood sugar was through the roof, and my body was showing all the classic signs of the cellular and organ damage that usually accompanies diabetes when it is untreated: I was exhausted, frequently sick, often hungry and more than 100 pounds overweight.

I quickly learned that this epidemic is largely self-inflicted. Most people diagnosed with diabetes are Type 2, meaning they have achieved their diabetic status through a combination of poor diet, little or no exercise, and a lifestyle that is all but certain to produce a diabetic diagnosis. Tens of millions of Americans have already been diagnosed with diabetes, and a similar number are already succumbing to the disease but have yet to be diagnosed, usually because they avoid seeing a physician, knowing that their physical condition and lifestyle choices are poor and are unlikely to result in any good news during a doctor's visit.

Diabetes is largely an environmental and lifestyle disease and one that is easily preventable, but a combination of factors, including our Western diet, high in processed foods and sugar, and a pharmaceutical and medical industry built around treating the disease rather than curing it, keeps the disease from killing us en masse but also fails to rid us of it or its debilitating effects. Those consequences are not just physical, but economic, and diabetics are now responsible in one way or another for nearly 20 percent of all health care costs in the United States.

The problem cannot be blamed solely on medical practitioners and their enablers in the pharmaceutical business; our entire agricultural and livestock industry, with the complicity of the

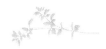

major food distributors, have filled store shelves with food that lasts longer, tastes sweeter, and looks brighter, but which is largely devoid of nutrition, and worse, may make you sick.

In their quest to construct foods that last longer, companies fill their products with preservatives. To build foods that look brighter, they use additives to brighten or change colors. To improve taste, they boost natural sugar levels with huge quantities of sugar (or worse, artificial sweeteners) or add huge amounts of salt. Many of the components in this process result in dangerous, toxic combinations that are alien to our bodies and contribute to the very factors that cause diabetes.

When I was diagnosed with diabetes, my physician prescribed a common drug for "managing" blood sugar: metformin. When one 850mg tablet per day didn't achieve the results, he increased the dose to two 850mg tablets a day. Eventually I was on three 850mg tablets daily to keep my blood sugar at an acceptable level. Sure enough, those levels remained static and my doctor was satisfied.

But as I evaluated my health, I saw that all the causes of my disease remained. I was overweight, which in itself was the result of too much of the wrong foods and a lack of exercise. I began relearning how to eat, recognizing that at thirty years old I could no longer eat like I had at age sixteen. I cut back on the pizza and fast food and started eating more salads. In a few months, I lost thirty pounds. Friends complimented me and I felt better, but to my surprise, I still needed to consume the same amount of metformin to keep the blood sugar counts at the right level.

Over time I grew accustomed to being diabetic and taking my medicine. I held my weight steady at about 235 pounds, down from nearly 280 pounds before I was diagnosed. But something new in my life awakened me to a new threat to my health: the possibility of a disruption to my supply of medicine and/or my easy access to my physician.

Off the Grid with Diabetes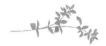

My parents had first introduced me to the concept of survivalism or "preparedness" in the run-up to the fears surrounding the 2000 computer "glitch" widely anticipated around the world. As 2000 passed without a catastrophe, interest in survivalism waned, but the idea remained in my own head.

In my profession I had grown accustomed to closely watching financial indicators and became worried about the direction of the economy. As the 2008 economic crisis came to fruition, it occurred to me that a complete collapse of the economy was not out of the realm of possibility and that the effects on society at large would be catastrophic. I began studying the results of economic collapse in other developed nations. I found the results to be horrifying: widespread unemployment, hyperinflation, and a breakdown of the government safety net almost always resulted in civil unrest, looting, rioting, and widespread violence.

At the same time I watched in dismay as the country elected a committed socialist to the highest office in the land. Obama has, to this time (early 2012), remained steadfast in his desire to implement European-style socialism in our country, beginning with the nationalization of our health care and the punishment of those who resist.

While studying these economic and political threats to our lifestyle, I became aware of other threats to our lifestyle including terrorism, natural disaster, war, a deteriorating infrastructure, and extraterrestrial threats, such as comets, asteroids, or solar events. As I explored the possible consequences on the financial markets of each of these potential events, I realized how fragile our society is and just how little it would take for our world to be seriously disrupted, and while the impact on our lives would be substantial from a stock market collapse, or hyperinflation, or a run on the bank, the impact on our health is far more grave. For example, if terrorists released a superbug that was designed to infect the masses and spread quickly, our health professionals would quickly be overwhelmed and unable to care for anyone

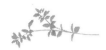

other than those most seriously ill (and who could pay). The youngest, oldest, sickest, and poorest would go to the back of the line. If you're suffering from a chronic disease, you may be out of luck. Worse, if the nation faces a real epidemic, the national security apparatus won't hesitate to quarantine you in your home until the crisis has passed. And if your medicine runs out—well, too bad.

The threats to your health don't hinge only on rare events like terrorist threats, however. Natural disasters, a collapsed bridge, or a single disruption at a factory across the world can lead to a shortage. Or, rolling blackouts may leave your local doctor or pharmacy unable to continue doing business. Of course, ever-rising prices threaten your pocketbook, and the difficult decision of what to do with ever fewer dollars is always present.

The story doesn't have to end badly though, regardless of how ominous the future may seem. I know just a few years ago at age thirty-four my health future didn't look so good; I had been diagnosed as diabetic years before, I had probably gone undiagnosed for years before that, and although my medicine kept the blood sugar in check, I knew that there were still long term threats to my life that could leave me blind and at risk of amputation, a life of pain, misery, and poor health, or even early death.

I decided I had had enough and made some changes. I spent a lot of time learning about food. I made some changes to my diet, and I developed a simple exercise routine that doesn't require a gym membership or any special equipment. I built a new diet around healthy, natural, sustainable foods and an exercise regime that I could conduct anywhere, anytime, regardless of my material possessions. I dropped another forty-five pounds and eliminated medication from my life. As I write this, I've not had my fasting blood sugar register more than ninety in almost two years, and I know how to eat, eat well, and enjoy food while avoiding those foods that can put my health at risk.

Off the Grid with Diabetes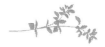

At the same time, I have accumulated the knowledge of how to treat my diabetes (I'll be diabetic for the rest of my life even if my blood sugar is under control) if and when I need treatment and do not have a medical professional and the entire pharmaceutical industry available to me.

What I discovered was the secret to living with and successfully treating diabetes beyond the reach of medicine where we all may find ourselves, whether because of a political environment that leaves us beyond the reach of medical professionals, a regulatory regime that decides who among the population is worthy of treatment, or an economic or infrastructure collapse that leaves those outside of the reach of urban medical facilities completely disconnected from modern medicine.

That is why I have written this book—to share with others who have suffered as I did with poor diet, a lack of exercise, and a debilitating disease the secret to overcoming all of these threats to your life and well being, and to remind you that the God who created everything has also supplied in nature the solutions to our problems.

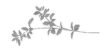

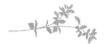

Chapter One:

Understanding Diabetes

Diabetes is a complex inflammatory disease that is often associated with high blood sugar, but diabetes is far more than just high blood sugar. Most experts believe that diabetes is the result of large amounts of free-radical damage—high levels of chemicals with resulting inflammation and nutritional deficiencies that can cause defective chemical pathways.

Some of the more complicated theories are that certain enzyme structures built into your genetic structure are to blame. However, virtually every expert agrees that diabetes is a metabolic disorder, and, for the majority of people, the disease can be managed through diet and exercise.

In our instant gratification society, we look to easy and quick solutions to complex problems, and the medical and pharmaceutical industry have satisfied that desire by prescribing medications for problems that can be solved naturally. Diabetes is a perfect example, because for the overwhelming number of diabetics, a regular exercise regime and a proper diet would rid them of the effects of the disease. Of course, for those who are not yet diabetic, but are suffering from some symptoms of the disease or who are on a trajectory for diagnosis, the same simple combination of diet and exercise can almost certainly reverse the effects.

However, once a person is on the road to a diabetic condition, their pancreas is being overwhelmed and their insulin levels begin to rise. Overtime, the pancreas begins to wear out and no longer functions as it should. Often times this is caused by little more than excess food intake.

It can be difficult to think about the pancreas and how it can become overworked, so an example may provide some insight.

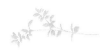 # Off the Grid with Diabetes

A healthy individual has a fasting level of glucose in his blood of approximately one teaspoon of sugar for every five quarts of blood. The consumption of something like a regular soda dumps ten to fifteen teaspoons of sugar into your body at one sitting. Imagine doing this several times over the course of the day, plus eating three meals and maybe a few snacks!

According to the American Diabetes Association, approximately 60 million Americans have hyperinsulinemia, hyperglycemia, or what is commonly referred to as insulin resistance. These conditions are referred to as pre-diabetes, which technically means a fasting blood sugar level between 100 and 125 milligrams per deciliter. At this stage, you don't really have Type 2 diabetes yet, but you're at great risk of developing it. The pre-diabetic is overworking his pancreas; insulin is being delivered to the body's cells, but the cells aren't accepting it, so the sugar remains in the bloodstream, wreaking havoc on your organs.

Your body recognizes that the cells aren't receiving the sugar they should, so the pancreas continues to manufacture insulin in increasing quantities, trying to force sugar into the cells, but the cells recognize the extra insulin and thus the process spirals out of control, usually leading to Type 2 diabetes. As the cells refuse the extra sugar and the insulin continues to build up, blood sugar levels rise above 125 mg/dl. When the body recognizes all this excess sugar, it tries to convert it into cholesterol and triglycerides for storage. But the extra cholesterol and triglycerides clog up your arteries, and of course the excessive sugar and insulin often lead to weight gain.

Type 2 diabetes is about more than just high blood sugar. The ripple effect throughout the body of the excess sugar floating around leads to all sorts of complications, including the inability of the body to deal with chemicals, leading to inflammation and organ failure or disruption, low levels of antioxidant production and problems with circulation. It truly is a case of the domino effect as one problem triggers a seemingly unending series of

Off the Grid with Diabetes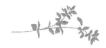

cascading and worsening health problems. For example, as sugar begins to build up in your blood, the body starts storing it in every nook and cranny it can—tiny capillaries all over your body, but particularly in blood-rich organs such as the kidneys, eyes, heart, and nerves. But just like any well-functioning machine, as all that material builds up, things don't work as well anymore. If the problem reaches the brain, it will stop recognizing and responding appropriately to signals from the rest of the body.

One such example is the "feel-full" hormone called leptin. Leptin's job is to tell your brain that you've eaten enough so you don't eat more than your body can process effectively. But if the brain is overwhelmed with sugar—literally floating in a sugar solution—it can't deal with this message and so, in a terrible irony, you never feel full. Thus, you'll continue eating, when it's most likely that overeating is contributing to this problem in the first place. That's why it's such a terrible disease and so hard for people who are diabetic and overweight, because the very way their body and brain are affected tends to perpetuate the diabetic cause. Eventually diabetes can lead to kidney failure, blindness, heart attack, stroke, and excruciating nerve pain.

A far more rare form of diabetes is known as Type 1 or juvenile-onset diabetes. I don't like the term "juvenile" because evidence indicates that many adults who are diagnosed as Type 2 are actually Type 1 sufferers, and diabetes Type 1 refers not to your age or the age of your diagnosis, but the inability of your pancreas to produce beta cells—the cells responsible for producing insulin. This is often the result of the body actually attacking the pancreas. Why this happens is still a matter of great debate, but the how is well understood.

Those suffering from Type 1 diabetes experience high levels of blood sugar because there is little or no insulin available to deliver sugar to the cells. Blood sugar therefore remains high unless insulin is provided to the body to deliver that sugar. Later in this

---

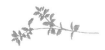

book, we will discuss natural alternatives to the artificial chemical insulin that most Type 1 diabetics become dependent upon.

There is another type of diabetes you've probably not heard of, known in the medical community as latent autoimmune diabetes in adults (LADA), or what some call Type 1.5 diabetes. This form of diabetes is the result of the body producing antibodies against its own pancreas. LADA requires constant insulin, unless you can determine why the antibodies are being generated in the first place. LADA is frustrating because it often occurs in people who have no behavioral traits normally associated with Type 2; they may be otherwise healthy, physically fit, and even eat a healthy diet.

One of the biggest problems in the diabetic community right now is the misdiagnosis of Type 1.5 as Type 2. There are tests of your c-peptide levels that can definitively determine whether you are Type 1.5 or Type 2, so if you have any questions, be sure to ask your doctor for this test. If you are Type 1.5 but are diagnosed as Type 2, you may initially respond to medication because your body will continue to produce some insulin, but as the disease progresses, your organs, especially the pancreas, will slowly fail until you become dependent on outside sources of insulin, by which time it may be too late to reverse the disease.

Because of the obesity epidemic in our culture, gestational diabetes is on the rise. This occurs in pregnant women who are overweight, and minorities tend to be at even greater risk. Gestational diabetes can be treated, but both mother and baby will remain at a higher risk of developing Type 2 for the rest of their lives. Just think of that poor baby being born into the world at risk of Type 2 diabetes just because of his mother's excess sugar intake (in most cases) during or before her pregnancy!

There is yet another type of diabetes—I know, the bad news never seems to stop—and it is called type 3 diabetes. Scientists have discovered a connection between people who have impaired

Off the Grid with Diabetes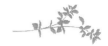

glucose metabolism and those with sluggish thinking. They've learned that the brain is also responsible for producing insulin in addition to the pancreas, further explaining the correlation between those with Type 2 diabetes and Alzheimer's disease. (The risk of Type 2 diabetics developing Alzheimer's is about 65 percent greater than the population at large).

In an odd twist, even though insulin resistance results in higher levels of blood sugar and insulin in the body, insulin levels in the brain actually fall. The brain stops functioning as well, and beta amyloids begin accumulating in unhealthy quantities. Fewer memory molecules are produced and as a result imbalances of even more critical brain chemicals are impaired, ultimately leading to cell damage. Talk about the domino effect!

This would be a good time to review some of the warning signs of diabetes. If you're anything like me, you'd rather have some advance warning about a life-threatening condition like diabetes. Finding out from your doctor in the cold impersonal exam room that you're one of the millions of undiagnosed diabetics walking around with what amounts to a ticking time bomb inside your blood is not an enjoyable experience. If you're educated, you can recognize the warning signs and begin to deal with it before it's too late.

When your brain is immersed in a sugar solution, it begins asking the body to supply it with fluid from any available source to dilute that concentrated sugar solution. As the brain is successful at pulling fluid from around the body, the cells that provided the fluid begin screaming for replacement, and the brain recognizes this as dehydration. In turn, it tells you that you're thirsty.

Unfortunately, many people respond by drinking something else sugary, like soda, which just compounds the problem by temporarily fooling you into thinking you're not thirsty while actually dumping more sugar into the bloodstream.

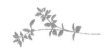 # Off the Grid with Diabetes

Of course, if you're drinking a lot and always feeling thirsty, it makes sense that you're going to be going to the bathroom a lot. This is because your kidneys are working overtime to pull extra water out of the bloodstream to dilute all the concentrated sugar, and so the floodgates open, filling up your bladder and telling you it's time to go to the bathroom. Of course, then the cycle starts all over again; you get thirsty, you drink more water to rehydrate, and the process continues until the excess glucose is eliminated. This cycle is a good and healthy thing if the glucose overload is a temporary problem, but over time the amount of protein that is being dumped into the urine by the kidneys interferes with its normal job of filtering the blood of wastes. This leads to toxins building up in your blood.

If you're feeling particularly weak or fatigued, what is now called chronic exhaustion, you might want to check your blood sugar. Sure, it's easy to have a cup of coffee or a soda or one of those energy drinks, but that's just dealing with symptoms, and we need to get to the cause!

When sugar from your meals can't get into your cells and provide them the energy source they need to function, you feel tired. Normally you would eat to gain energy, but in this case, your eating is the problem, not the solution, and this kind of tiredness isn't cured by sleep. And yet, your body is so confused at this point that the starving cells will actually tell your body they are hungry for food, confusing you further and giving you that sense that you can't get full. You might also feel like you need to sleep all the time. Sometimes people confuse this desire to eat and sleep with depression, but just because you're feeling bad about being overweight and tired and hungry all the time doesn't mean you're clinically depressed!

One of the worst consequences of diabetes is nerve damage, which can take years to develop. The medical term for this is neuropathy, which develops when your bloodstream is overwhelmed by glucose. Excess glucose can sometimes act

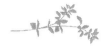

like an acid on your nerves by damaging the tiny, delicate, and fragile nerve endings that are found in your extremities. You start to feel pain, numbness, tingling, itching, and other strange sensations. If this happens, you need to discuss it immediately with your physician.

As we discussed earlier, dehydration is a common result of high blood sugar, and the brain will pull fluid from all possible locations in your body, including your eyes, where fluid is stored in the lenses, giving you the ability to focus. In addition, the capillaries in your eyes that control movement and focus can become damaged by all the free radicals that are floating around.

It's easy to understand why the lenses of your eyes are so important—clear vision is critical to life— and those awful free radicals are harmful molecules that must be dealt with. Nature's solution is antioxidants, because they neutralize the effects of free radicals. We'll talk about natural sources of antioxidants later, but if you notice any change in your vision, be sure to see your doctor immediately.

Another sign of insulin resistance is a skin condition known as acanthosis nigricans, which appears as patches of dark skin in the folds and creases of the body. You might notice this discoloration: it looks like dirt in the armpit, neck, groin, and knuckles.

If you begin to notice that you are experiencing frequent or prolonged infections, particularly bladder or vaginal infections, it might be a sign of your body's inability to resist or naturally heal. Antibiotics may no longer have the curative effect they do in a healthy person because the body itself is so weakened. Combine this with the growing occasions of antibiotic resistance in the population, and you have a truly dangerous environment for infection.

One of the more unusual signs of diabetes is losing weight without really trying. Remember, when the cells aren't getting the sugar

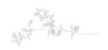

they need, they can't produce the energy your body needs, and as a result your muscles feel famished. The diabetic responds by snacking constantly, and yet occasionally this person will suddenly start losing weight! You might be thinking, "Wow, I can eat all the time and still lose weight!"

Unfortunately, this kind of weight loss is extremely dangerous, because your body is actually converting muscle into energy, literally eating itself in order to feed the cells' demand for energy.

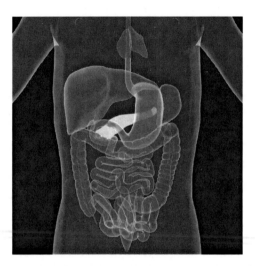

This is more common in Type 1 diabetes, because Type 2 diabetics tend to be overweight and so the weight loss is more easily disguised. However, any weight loss that is unexplained or runs counter to your lifestyle should be a source of concern, not joy.

Regardless of the type of diabetes or blood sugar disorder we consider, we need to understand the risk factors. Fortunately this disease is so widely studied we have a great understanding of the factors.

First, the older you are, the greater your risk for developing diabetes, whether you're slim or fat. The reason for this is the accumulated consequences of free radical damage to your cells, particularly those in your pancreas.

If you're overweight, as nearly two thirds of all Americans are, you are at a much greater risk of developing diabetes. In fact, it's the number one predictor of diabetes because in most cases the overweight person is eating more than their body can healthily

Off the Grid with Diabetes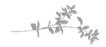

use and convert into energy, the very same problem that we see at the cellular level.

Similarly, if you're not getting enough exercise, you may find yourself in a situation where it is very easy to consume more sugar than your body can convert to energy. If you exercise you are increasing the number of muscle cells in your body, thereby increasing the number of insulin receptors, making it a lot easier for your body to convert sugar into energy.

Fat cells don't have that extra ability to deal with the insulin and sugar, so as you pile on fat cells, you are compounding the problem. Exercise, on the other hand, also causes your insulin to work more effectively because your cells are actually demanding more of it, not less. Studies have shown that as little as one hour of exercise per week starts the process of increasing beta cell function and insulin sensitivity. This may sound complicated, but it's actually really simple in practice, and later in the book I will provide some methods of exercise that anyone can do, anywhere, without joining a gym or buying weights or getting into expensive or dangerous workout regimes.

A lot of Americans are couch potatoes. Most have learned this behavior from their parents, and if you have a parent or sibling who is Type 2, watch out! Doctors have discovered that family members are at a greater risk too, not because the disease is contagious, but because lifestyles are learned at a very early age. Therefore, if you learn to eat a certain way and develop lethargic life habits from your parents, and then they develop Type 2 diabetes, the odds are pretty good that you will too. If you see someone you are close to develop the disease, check your own health for these risk factors.

So far we've talked around the disease, but before we move on, we need to spend just a few moments on the critical body organs that are affected by this disease. I know, you didn't sign up for a biology course, but there may come a day when you don't have

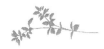

access to a doctor or the Internet to research how your body works (or doesn't), and having this knowledge in your head may save a life one day:

Your body has two types of glands, endocrine and exocrine, and their job is to secrete substances that include enzymes, hormones, and metabolites. In addition to the pancreas, the thyroid, hypothalamus, pituitary gland, adrenals, and even fat cells are endocrine glands, and they all produce hormones. The pancreas' primary job is regulating blood sugar and digesting food, which is why it is so central to the diabetic disorder.

During digestion, your body relies on two hormones, incretin and insulin, to break down and regulate sugar in your body. When they work together properly, they reduce stress on the pancreas and actually help to reduce fat and cholesterol throughout your body.

The pancreas is also responsible for digestion-related enzymes, which help to break food particles into tiny molecules that are more easily digested. As the pancreas is doing this, it creates insulin, which is simply a delivery method for getting sugar to the cells. As we've already discussed, if the sugar is present in your body but not being accepted by the cells, your blood sugar spikes. Conventional medicine uses artificial chemicals to deal with insulin resistance, but we're going to be exploring natural ways to correct the problem rather than merely treat the symptom.

Someone once described insulin as a password that tells your cells to open and accept sugar. When you're healthy, the pancreas recognizes the level of insulin in the blood and adapts. But if the insulin can't get the cells to accept your sugar, then it floats around in the body, doing damage. The old expression "idle hands are the devil's handiwork" is a good way of thinking about that idle sugar; it was meant to supply cells with energy, and when it can't do that, it's like a toddler full of energy left alone at home for a day. Only bad things happen! In fact, when all this sugar has

---

Off the Grid with Diabetes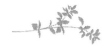

been floating around your system, all sorts of problems occur. Diabetics frequently experience B vitamin deficiencies, mineral deficiencies, imbalanced stomach acids, reduced adrenal performance, thyroid impairment, liver dysfunction, and colon toxicity. Most diabetic treatments ignore these compounding failures and simply try to manage the high blood sugar. In this book we'll explore natural treatments of the underlying causes and how you can reverse the effects.

Many discussions of diabetes ignore a common problem that should be mentioned. Fungal infections are common problems that accompany diabetes. We all have fungi living in our bodies, and researchers believe fungi counts may be as much as 3 percent of our total microbial count. They are everywhere: on our skin, in our mouth, in our intestines, on our hair, and in our urinary tract. We cannot live without them, but we also need them to be in balance.

Fungus feeds on sugar, and an overabundance of sugar in the body can stimulate yeast and fungi production and tip this otherwise healthy system into overproduction, leading to fungal infection. Some studies have shown that as little as two extra teaspoons of sugar a day can lead to fungal growth in the body! Just imagine what a few sodas, several alcoholic beverages, a sugary candy, or a rich dessert contains!

To fungi and yeast, insulin is an enemy; therefore, fungi create toxins that are hostile to insulin. In the diabetic, insulin resistance is already an issue, so a fungal infection presents a serious threat, and yet, fungal infections, particularly within organs, are extremely difficult to diagnose. Worse, fungi create dangerous micro-toxins that are poisonous to your organs and can slowly kill them. Your body may already be laboring under an abundance of sugar, a brain that isn't working properly, a pancreas that is overwhelmed, and now a growth of fungus! You've probably heard of **Candida Albicans**, a scientific name for that notorious yeast which, in the extreme, can lead to a yeast infection; in your

---

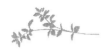

organs, this kind of yeast infection can seriously impair your organ function, and worse, the food you are eating may actually promote these organ yeast infections.

What kind of foods might promote this growth? I'm sorry to say that some of my favorites (and probably yours) are on the list: pasta, bread, crackers, cereals, cookies, bagels, white sauces, gravies, and pastries! But all is not lost. In the next chapter we'll begin exploring exactly how and why these foods are hurting you and what you can do to eat great and still avoid diabetes (or reverse it!)

Chapter Two:

Your Diet is Killing You

The diabetic epidemic has exploded in the Western world as diets have changed from largely whole-food based food intake to diets based on commercially processed, store-bought foods high in starch and sugars. These foods, now dominating the diets of Europe and the Americas, are high in chemicals and additives necessary to survive the long and often hostile environment necessary to get food from the commercial farms and laboratories to the grocery shelves near the consumer.

One hundred years ago, most Americans lived and worked on farms and grew a portion of their food. That which they did not grow, they traded for or purchased from other local farmers. Virtually their entire diet was based on locally grown, naturally prepared, nutritious food. Today, the reverse is true; only 2 percent of Americans work on farms, and the overwhelming majority of the food we consume is purchased through huge multinational food conglomerates whose job is to prepare and package food that looks good, tastes good, and lasts a long time on the shelves (and in transport conditions where temperature ranges are extreme.)

In order to accomplish this feat, food processors and distributors fabricate foods that employ artificial flavorings, preservatives, and dyes. All these things help the food look better than it otherwise would, appear fresh even when there is an underlying deterioration taking place, and give you that initial burst of flavor, sweetness, or saltiness that causes your brain to think, "Wow, this is really good."

In order to boost yields over that which is normal to nature (and to therefore increase corporate profitability), agriculture businesses have also turned to genetically modifying foods to create an entirely new "species" of food. The publicly stated purpose is to produce foods that are more resistant to bacteria and pests, and while this is certainly part of their objective, a basic understanding of economics and mankind also reinforces that these mega-corporations won't act in a way that is counter to their financial interest. As a result, genetically modified foods may grow bigger, appear brighter, and have more intense flavor than their natural counterparts. That they are also largely void of nutrition is a little-known secret in the industry.

A very high percentage of the food we buy from the store contains genetically engineered components in one form or another. Many of these components have never been proven safe for human consumption. In fact, in testing among rats, genetically modified corn has led to atrophy of internal organs and may be a contributor to organ failure and diabetes. Arpad Pusztai tested genetically engineered potatoes and found that the animals developed organ damage, particularly in the pancreas, which we know is central to the regulation of insulin. Among the foods in our society that are most likely to contain genetic modifications are soy, corn, cotton-seed, potatoes, and commercial milk products.

To understand just how bad most of the food we buy at the store is, we need to get back to basics. We eat in order to survive. Food provides nourishment for our cells. Our cells contain no artificial additives, and they prefer food that is free of artificial components. They work best at absorbing nutrients that are familiar to the human body—chemicals that have been a part of our diet for tens of thousands of years. And yet, today's commercial products contain huge quantities of synthetic food dyes, food flavorings, aspartame, synthetic vitamins, inorganic iron, propylene glycol, and MSG. These additives don't provide additional nutritional value, but they do add to the shelf life of the products, allowing the manufacturers to build logistical lines that are longer and more profitable. If a tomato normally deteriorates and rots in a week, but a commercial farm can pump that same tomato full of chemicals that make it bigger and redder and lasts for a full month, it is easy

Off the Grid with Diabetes

to see why said corporation will do it, but the question of whether the tomato is safe for human consumption remains.

If you're anything like me, you are no doubt wondering, "Well don't we have the FDA for that?" If we assume for a moment that the FDA—a government body—can be trusted to protect our interests (and I would suggest that is one very big assumption), then we have to wonder how it is we can be so certain that something is safe when its use in human nutrition is a revolutionary and new development. What if it takes a full generation for the impact of these chemicals to manifest themselves? What if the consequences don't show up until late in life? Does that mean we are subject to an entire generation of experimentation?

What if, for example, all these chemicals and additives contribute to the development of Alzheimer's disease, something that usually shows up very late in life (and is largely untreatable)? That Alzheimer's was a relatively unknown disease until the most recent generation is indisputable. That the use of chemicals and additives was largely unheard of until the most recent generation is also indisputable. The correlation doesn't prove that all these artificial additives cause Alzheimer's, but the burden of proof on any novelty—especially one critical to life and health— should be on the novelty. I suggest that we should experiment over long periods of time—with humans, not rats—before exposing the entire population to unproven and possibly dangerous additives.

Commercial testers and those who supply data to the FDA and big business will say that rats share most of our genetic data and reproduce quickly, therefore giving us a reliable indicator of what these additives will do in humans over several generations. Of course, rats are also cheaper to study than humans. That testing agencies are concerned about cost can be no surprise to any reader, and that a government agency will rely on an outside source for data that it can then use to justify a political decision is also likely to surprise no one. Remember how the FHA, Fannie, Freddie, and the entire mortgage banking business relied on a

---

few bureaucrats at the rating agencies (privately held, for-profit businesses) to determine the risk of mortgage securities? That political and profit motive led to the liquidity crisis of 2008 and almost brought the world economy to a standstill.

One premise of this book is that we cannot trust the government or big business to protect our interests. We can expect that they will protect THEIR interests. That doesn't mean that they're out to poison us, but it does mean that first and foremost they are concerned with what is good for them. Keeping that in mind, we should carefully evaluate whatever we hear from Wall Street or Washington and filter it through the healthy skepticism of a Christian who understands the fallen nature of man.

I believe that diabetes is caused in many cases by a lack of healthy, nutritious food. I know, you're thinking that diabetes is caused by eating too much food—but what if that is a symptom rather than a cause? What if people are eating food that doesn't really provide their cells the nutrition they need to properly function, and as a result the body screams out for more food, so the person responds by eating even more, and a terrible cycle quickly develops?

This is known as starvation syndrome, where cells fail to get sufficient nutrients. Without the key ingredients the cells need, such as vitamins, minerals, essential fatty acids, enzymes, and amino acids, the cells start to get sick. When they are sick, they can't function and begin to die. If these cells that are sick or dying are located in your skin, then your skin isn't as healthy and you might notice dry or inelasticity or poor appearance. If the dying cells are in your eyes, your eyesight might fail. If the dying cells are in your organs, then organs fail. A pancreas that is failing might have trouble producing or regulating the insulin. See a pattern?

Another theory that is gaining in credibility among experts and nutritionists is that as these chemicals build up in the body, toxicity levels reach highs that cannot be adequately dealt with

Off the Grid with Diabetes

by the body. These poisons will naturally build up in key organs that normally detoxify the body, such as the pancreas, liver, and kidneys. It doesn't take much toxicity to see deterioration in organ performance, and it's not hard to see how someone whose lifestyle has led them to depend almost entirely on ready-to-eat meals, fast food, or packaged junk food finds themselves starving, so they eat more. In the meantime, their cells continue to scream for more, they gain weight while starving themselves, and those chemicals that make all that food appear good, taste good, and last on the shelf start to cause organ failure. Pretty soon the consumer is fat, sick, feeling terrible, and on his way to a diabetic diagnosis.

The link between diabetes and diet is well known. As early as the first century A.D., Hippocrates theorized that the over-consumption of alcohol and sweets led to this disease. At the same time, physicians in India had identified the cause of this disease as being obesity brought on by a sedentary lifestyle and too much sugar.

Ten centuries later in Persia, the famous scientist Ibn Sina discovered that the urine of diabetics had a sweet smell and that non-diabetic urine did not. He made the obvious connection that diabetics had too much sugar in their body and that this must come from too much consumption. Our own easy observation today shows that most diabetics eat too much and eat poorly.

In our own era, we can look at populations that are largely insulated from the modern Western-style diet and find a very low incidence of diabetes. Among the Inuit living in a native society, diabetes is extremely rare, although they eat a diet high in fat. However, among the Inuit who have moved into civilization and adopted a typical Western diet, a very high rate of diabetes is common. Scientists have speculated that an Inuit who has no previous tolerance of our complex foods cannot deal with all the additives and therefore responds more quickly and adversely than

---

someone who has spent their entire life exposed to the same toxins. Kind of scary, isn't it?

A similar phenomenon has been observed with other native peoples. The Yemeni Jews, with a diet rich in whole milk products, butterfat, and red meat, are generally free of diabetes, but once exposed to the Western diet, they develop a very high incidence of diabetes, as do American Pima Indians. Among the Misaim tribe of Africa, diabetes in nature is a rare event, occurring in 1 of 300 individuals, but again, under the influence of the Western diet, diabetes will suddenly manifest itself in 1 in 10, a rate 30 times higher!

We see the same trend among non-native peoples. In the early part of the last century, diabetes was a rare disease affecting only a small segment of people—the rich who had access to unlimited quantities of alcohol and rare sugar-based sweets.

However, as trade developed and refined sugar began to make its way into the diet of the Western world and the mass production of sweets and better distribution methods brought these products into the average home, the incidence of diabetes grew exponentially. By the 1930s, average sugar consumption had risen dramatically, and by the 1960s, diabetes was being referred to as an epidemic. Since the first introduction of refined sugar into the mass population 100 years ago, sugar consumption has increased 100 fold. The effect has been disastrous.

Refined sugar calories displace the otherwise healthy intake of food. On its own, sugar is not doing anything good for the body, while at the same time, it tends to prevent the intake of good food. In the United States prior to World War II, the average American consumed about twenty pounds of sugar per year; by the 1970s, that had increased to 100 pounds, and by the year 2000, the average rate of consumption was an astonishing 150 pounds of sugar! That's three pounds per week! That sugar brings about horrific health consequences is easily determined

Off the Grid with Diabetes

by comparing the sugar intake in poor countries and the corresponding lower rates of diabetes. They simply can't afford to import the processed, refined sugar that makes them sick!

When we consider the obesity epidemic among children in the West, we can easily identify the culprit. Children love to eat sweets, and parents, grandparents, caregivers, and the industry are generally happy to fill that demand. In previous generations, the sugar was either unavailable or unaffordable. The average consumption of sugar by American children now exceeds 200 pounds per year. The effects on a growing mind and body, still desperate for nutrients, are devastating. Sugar-related diseases include hypoglycemia, eczema, asthma, juvenile arthritis, tooth decay, leukemia, anxiety, depression, schizophrenia, attention deficit, autism, and cancer.

As the build up in the body of sugar displaces other nutrients and bathes the organs in sugar concentrate, the body stops working as efficiently. As a result, many of these children lack key vitamins and minerals for insulin synthesis. Deficiencies of zinc, copper, chromium, vitamin C, vitamin B6, thiamine, niacin, and pantothenic acid are common.

Sugar is a relatively new ingredient in the human diet. It is also completely devoid of nutritional value. This is not to say that natural sugar, such as that found in maple syrup, honey, or fruit is not nutritious, because these natural sources are high in minerals, potassium and even vitamin C. But refined sugar is 99.9 percent nutrient free, a pure carbohydrate that robs the body of nutrients.

In the past, mankind used natural honey as a sweetener, and there was no corresponding increase in diabetes. However, once sugar cane entered the diet during the Victorian era and was further refined, men became addicted, and the demand has increased ever since. As use in food products has increased over the last century, new diseases have developed, dental decay has exploded, and heart disease, arthritis, and cancer have become commonplace.

It is important to understand why this refined sugar is so bad for us, so we can properly apply the concept to our new way of living; in fact, an off-the-grid form of living will almost guarantee we are free of the diabetic threat.

Sugar in its natural form is full of minerals, which give it a dark, almost dirty color. In order to create a pure white appearance, the nutrient rich juices are squeezed out of the cane sugar and the beet sugar is entirely eliminated. Next, lime or carbon dioxide is added in order to further cleanse the sugar of minerals, vitamins, and flavonoids. Then the sugar is heated to an extremely high temperature to generate the consistency that manufacturers desire. In the process, any remaining nutritional value is completely eliminated. But the process is far from complete, because phosphoric acid and milk of lime are added to oxidize the sugar to a pure white color, consistent with what Western consumers have been told to expect from sugar. Then, in order to remove any remaining protein sugars, they actually bathe the remaining substance with hog and cattle albumin, which binds with the naturally recurring protein and further refines it. The result is a glimmering white bleached powder that is available for commercial sale. It is also now a fully artificial creation with no nutritional value and no place in our diet.

The nutrition industry long ago developed alternatives to sugar, recognizing the dangers of refined sugar, but these alternatives aren't much better. Saccharin is created from the residue left over from the heating of coal within gas plants. This noxious, black tar substance is a byproduct that is dangerous for human consumption, and yet it is now the raw material used for synthesizing chemicals, both in food and in drugs, because it is so effective at bonding molecules. Although it was once banned as a food additive (and still is in Canada), it is now back in American diets.

Off the Grid with Diabetes

Aspartame, a popular alternative, has a similarly ugly history. It is a chemical consisting of amino acids plus a substance similar to methanol, the dangerous component of moonshine. Researchers studying the chemistry of aspartame have shown that when ingested, it is broken down into amino acids and methanol, the toxicity of which is well known. In fact, in the lab methanol is labeled with a skull and crossbones, and yet many beverages are laced with it!

While sugar is the primary culprit in our modern diets, unfortunately, it is not the only one. Americans consume on average about twenty-two gallons of milk yearly, and that milk is largely contaminated. In April of 2004, **Hoard's Dairyman**, the magazine of the National Dairy Farms, revealed that milk contains about 750 million pus cells per liter. Other studies found that a liter of milk also contained traces of blood, mucus, feces, and dangerous microorganisms.

If you think about it, the fact that we drink cow's milk at all is a little unusual. We're the only mammals that drink any milk after infancy, let alone milk from a totally different species. You would expect a calf to drink cow's milk, but not a human baby (we have human milk for that, after all). But we do drink lots of milk, and cow's milk is processed and turned into a wide variety of other dairy items, such as cream, butter, cheese, yogurt, and ice cream. The threat from milk is so great that even the American Academy of Pediatrics, which used to whole-heartedly recommend whole milk, eventually suggested that toddlers should be weaned off whole milk. Then they reduced that recommendation in 2008 to children age two. Then they further changed their recommendation, saying anyone who is at risk of being overweight or has a history of obesity, heart disease, or high cholesterol should not drink whole milk.

Then the Academy suggests that after twelve months of age, no one should drink anything other than 1 percent milk! And yet the industry continues to fund studies that selectively show

---

the benefits of milk. And yet no fewer than eleven different clinical studies have shown a link between whole milk consumption in children and diabetes. In fact, Type 1 diabetes is the most common form of diabetes in many parts of the world, especially among children. And, the highest prevalence of Type 1 diabetes in children is found in areas that also are known for a higher rate of consumption of cow's milk: Finland, Sweden, Norway, and Great Britain. Where consumption of cow's milk is lowest, the incidence of Type 1 diabetes is also lowest; for example, in China it is found at a rate of 0.1 cases per 100,000 infants, where in Finland it is 37 per 100,000, an enormous increase!

In fact, the risk is so great that the **Journal of Pediatric Diabetes** lists the consumption of cow's milk at an early age as a risk factor along with C-section delivery, stomach viruses in the mother, and preeclampsia. There might not be much that can be done about a necessary C-section, but surely we can alter our voluntary consumption of pus-laden cow's milk!

So how exactly is cow's milk so dangerous? As babies are weaned off of their mother's milk and onto cow's milk, the milk proteins are ingested by the intestine and proteins such as casein are digested as amino acids. But for many infants, this foreign milk is not fully digested, and so some food globules are absorbed into the bloodstream. The immune system recognizes these foreign "invaders" and begins trying to kill the foreign proteins. Unfortunately, these proteins happen to look a lot like beta cells in the baby's pancreas, and the immature immune system has a hard time distinguishing between the two. The introduction of these foreign cow's milk cells therefore tricks the immune system into destroying the pancreas, and once accomplished, the child can no longer produce insulin. Type 1 diabetes is born.

Unfortunately, it's not as easy as eliminating milk from the diet because food manufacturers are so good at producing other products from milk.

Off the Grid with Diabetes

When milk is made into cheese, whey protein is a byproduct. It is commonly used as a supplement in many ice creams, smoothies, and milk shakes. Whey supplements are also found in body building products because they contain the amino acid cysteine, which in its natural form is a powerful antioxidant.

Powdered milk is also popular and is commonly used in infant supplements. The problem is that powdered milk usually contains oxysterols, which are free radicals that can lead to a clogging of the arteries. Sweetened condensed milk is just cow's milk that has had the water removed and sugar added. This sweet concoction is used in dessert recipes and can stay fresh for years. That alone should be a warning sign!

Because milk has to be pasteurized in order to kill dangerous microorganisms, many of the healthy enzymes and vitamins are also killed. It's a classic case of throwing the baby out with the bathwater. Along with pasteurization comes the destruction of vitamin C and iodine, and calcium often times becomes insoluble. Raw milk is clearly more nutritious for you, but because of the higher risk of bacterial infection from salmonella, listeria, and fecal contamination, no large dairy producer wants to run the risk of litigation. The result is a milk product that contains far fewer benefits and far more dangerous chemical additives. For most Americans, this means a higher risk of weak bones, bad teeth, and infections because the calcium can't be absorbed.

Another problem with cow's milk is the prominent protein casein. It's also found in many soy products. Casein in the body turns into casomorphin, which results in the release of histamine. Histamine is what you would commonly associate with allergies and asthma, but in this case it can also lead to diabetes. Have you ever noticed someone sneeze after eating foods that contain a dairy product? Those who have allergy or asthma problems can usually adopt a dairy-free diet and see an immediate improvement in their symptoms.

Unfortunately casein is not the only culprit here, as lactose also presents problems. Lactose is a sugar found in raw milk, and when we're very young, we have a lot of lactase to help our body break down lactose. However, as we age, we quickly lose our supply of lactase and therefore our ability to process the lactose in milk. The problem is that as milk is pasteurized, the lactose becomes a sugar that is more easily absorbed into the bloodstream, meaning that you become hungrier faster because you're not as easily satisfied. You may be so lacking in lactase that you become completely lactose intolerant. The symptoms are digestive problems, ranging from cramps and rumbling in your stomach to loose stools, constipation, gas, bloating, and nausea. Unfortunately, milk and milk by-products are also found in many caramel colors, naturalose (often used as a low calorie sweetener in foods), drinks, candies, energy bars, toothpaste, mouthwash, canned tuna fish, chicken broth, and wine (where it is used to remove impurities).

All this talk about milk is important because if you are already susceptible to diabetes, putting the additional strain on your body is not a wise idea, and anything that further complicates your organ efficiency can push you over the line into a diabetic diagnosis. A particularly bad allergy to milk can lead to catastrophic organ breakdown, which can then trigger diabetes as insulin production is disrupted. A simple thing like milk! And yet as we have learned it's a foreign food supply to our bodies and probably shouldn't be there in the first place. We'll talk more about alternative foods later, but for your quick reference, good substitutes for cow's milk include goat, almond, rice, hemp, and oat milk. They are far better choices.

I know that I've been delivering a lot of bad news, but unfortunately, I've got some more. Milk isn't the only unusual product that your body isn't really designed for that probably forms some part of your diet. Bread is also a prime suspect as a trigger of diabetes. Now, before you throw your hands up in exasperation at another favorite food item that may well be slowly killing you, let me make the case and share some strategies for healthy living (and enjoyment).

Bread has long been a staple of the human diet, but the bread you buy at the store today bears little resemblance to what our ancestors made (or what our Lord used to feed the thousands). Today's commercial farmers apply a huge amount of pesticides to the food to protect the crop. As we discussed earlier, we can understand why the farmer would want to use pesticide (it helps him generate more revenue than if crop was lost to disease), but are these pesticides good for us? Well, unfortunately, eighty-three of the active ingredients in pesticides still in use today are harmful to us (and have been shown in clinical studies to cause cancer in animals).

Once that grain has been harvested and placed in a grain elevator, it sits in an environment that is dark and often warm, leading to a potential growth of fungus. The primary threat to us is **Fusarium Graminearum**, a fungus that can cause vomiting, diarrhea, skin problems, and immune suppression. In the old days, wheat wasn't stored as long or as frequently, and so the risk from fungi was greatly reduced, but today's wheat market is so massive and efficient

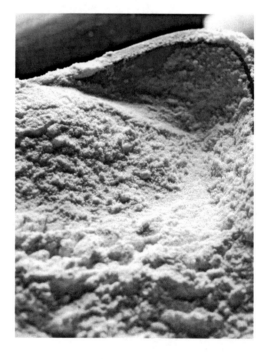

that grain operators will time their storage to maximize profit, often meaning that wheat will sit for months and sometimes years if future prices are anticipated to be higher than current market prices. The longer the wheat sits and the greater the temperature variation, the greater the potential for fungal growth.

Most wheat is then ground into flour, and most of this is all-purpose flour. In order to create all-purpose flour, the wheat kernels are stripped of their bran and germ layers, which removes the most nutritious parts of the grain. What is lost in this process is the fiber, minerals, and vitamins that are naturally occurring and help make wheat so nutritious. Although the very best part of the grain has been removed, the flour will now command a higher price in the market because of the greater processing required to get it to this stage. Because the wheat is naturally brown, and the market favors white flour, chlorine gas will be used to bleach the flour. Of course, chlorine gas is dangerous to inhale and is irritating to the human body, even lethal in some circumstances, and yet it is part of the process of manufacturing all-purpose flour.

When chlorine gas comes into contact with the wheat, one of the byproducts is a toxin called alloxan. Alloxan looks similar to glucose at the molecular level and is often mistaken by the body as glucose.

In fact, alloxan is such a good disguise for glucose that in clinical tests, scientists use alloxan to test the damage on organ function. It is so effective that when scientists want to study pancreatic failure in lab rodents, they inject alloxan!

Not every flour manufacturer creates alloxan as part of their process, but many do. If you are eating a lot of products made from white flour, as most Americans do, then the odds are you are consuming a fair amount of alloxan.

According to the Textbook of Natural Medicine, alloxan is a "potent beta-cell toxin." The long-term ingestion of alloxan can put you at risk for diabetes and all of its complications, including coma, amputation, blindness, kidney failure, nerve pain, and of course, death.

Off the Grid with Diabetes

Regrettably, the bad news about commercially produced bread doesn't end with alloxan. Gluten, which helps to hold bread together, is another health risk. Gluten is found in many types of bread including wheat, rye, barley, spelt, and kamut. Of course, all-purpose flour comes from wheat, so this is a primary carrier of gluten. If you have a gluten allergy (and you may not even know it, as the symptoms are often misdiagnosed), you could be setting up your body to become more susceptible to organ deterioration and ultimately diabetes.

Remember that people with Type 1 diabetes and gluten sensitivities have a higher prevalence of autoimmune thyroid disease. If your thyroid is responding by producing antibodies (something your physician can easily measure), then you know that you have a problem with gluten. Of course, thyroid function is linked to diabetes, because as you relieve stress on your organs, their ability to deal with insulin and glucose is improved and your risk of diabetes is greatly diminished.

At the same time, if you have a sensitivity to gluten, and many people do, you're putting a great deal of stress on your digestive system, inhibiting the proper absorption of nutrients that your cells need to properly function. We've already reviewed how this failure to properly feed your cells can lead to a cascade of problems that can result in diabetes.

I recognize that milk and bread products form the core of much of the Western diet and many of our favorite foods. At the same time, we have already seen how it is our very diet that is bringing about the health epidemic we have, so some kind of change is necessary.

The unexpected silver lining here is that the very source of our problems—commercially prepared food products that are dangerous to our health—are the same problems we can overcome as we prepare for an off-the-grid lifestyle. We CAN enjoy dairy products that are not dependent on commercial producers who have their profit motives ahead of our health, and we CAN enjoy bread products that don't carry dangerous chemicals that threaten our health.

The solutions are there for us; all we need to do is return to time-honored, proven methods of growing healthy crops and raising livestock close to the demand for food and in a way that the consumer (you and I) can judge its safety for ourselves. The problem is not the free market, but a corporatist version of capitalism that places big business in partnership with big government to maximize profits, maximize regulation and reward those politicians who protect the interests of both, and it all depends on a submissive population that is ignorant of the consequences. Together we can change that system.

Chapter Three:

Big Pharma

Big pharmaceutical companies (Big Pharma) and your doctors want to treat you, not heal you. As we've already discussed in previous chapters, whenever you engage in commerce, it's wise to remember that the other party in the transaction has motives of their own which are likely not the same as yours. That's not to say they are counter to your interests, but only that each man (or corporation or government) protects its own interests.

Big Pharma has its own interests. First and foremost, they exist to generate profits for their shareholders and big salaries, bonuses, and benefits for their management teams. They also must have sufficient margins to employ the teams of six and seven-figure lobbyists who roam the halls of Congress and wine and dine the federal regulatory agencies that approve and manage the regulation of new and modified pharmaceutical products. Without profits, none of those things are possible. It's not that profits are evil—quite the contrary—but in a secular society such as ours, where a corporation by law has only a profit motive, and acknowledges no obligation to man or God, then it is natural that a corporation will put that one end (or objective) above all others.

It should be apparent that Big Pharma wants to sell drugs. The only way to generate profits is through the development of drugs that provide benefits to the consuming public. In order to develop these drugs the companies need to conduct massive amounts of research, which is often very expensive. There is countless research and experimentation involved in finding and testing the complex combination of chemicals and biological agents in order to find drugs that achieve the desired outcome without (too many) harmful side effects. A lot of mice die in the process, and the right kind of mice aren't cheap either!

Off the Grid with Diabetes

Drug companies won't fund just any research though; as profit-motivated capitalists, they have lots of different options for spending their capital, and they reasonably want to do so in a way that will achieve the greatest possible return on their investment (ROI). If a research team discovers that one combination of chemicals costs "X" and achieves 80 percent success, but another costs "2X" and achieves 85 percent success, good economics would suggest the former is a better investment.

We reach that conclusion because the improvement in efficacy is less than 10 percent while the cost is increased by 100 percent. This is a common phenomenon in medicine by the way, where we reach the point of diminishing returns, where the gains are offset by vastly greater costs. However, because the American public believes it is entitled to the very best of anything, the market, perversely, is willing to pay for "the best" (who wants to have the "second best" treatment?), and so the drug companies are more than willing to invest in products that are only marginally better than another, even if the cost is dramatically greater.

Why?

The drug companies are just going to pass those costs along. It doesn't really matter to them what the raw cost is, because their overhead is so great that it is largely fixed, so to use an accounting term, the variable costs of the actual drugs manufactured is just passed along, with the appropriate markup. In fact, in the end, the drug company makes far more money on an expensive drug. If drug A costs $20 to make and the drug company marks it up 300 percent, it sells for $60 and they make $40. But if the drug costs $100 and they mark it up 300 percent, it sells for $300. It's the same markup—you can't allege any sort of discriminatory pricing—but the net impact on the bottom line is dramatic. Instead of booking $40 in net income, the management gets to book $200 in net income—an increase of 500 percent!

Off the Grid with Diabetes

Keeping in mind that management is driven by two primary interests— first, preserving their lucrative salaries and generating the largest possible bonuses (which almost always are tied to profitability or share price) and second, generating share gains (when the price of a stock goes up shareholders are happy) or generating dividends, which can only be paid if there are profits! So it's easy to see why management, which is the decision maker day-to-day, would choose to bring to market a more expensive drug, even if it is only marginally better.

You might be thinking that insurance companies, since they pay the bills for most medicine, would kind of be watchdogs on this and have an incentive to keep the costs low. But you'd be wrong. The insurance companies don't really care what the drugs cost, because they're just passing those costs along as well. How so? Well, the only reason they provide insurance coverage is because someone is paying premiums, and those premiums are established based on the expected cost of providing coverage over the term that is covered.

The way insurance works is the company looks at a huge pool of similar people, say for example, diabetics. They aggregate all the normal costs of providing medical care to a Type 2 diabetic, from the doctor's visit to the likelihood of emergency care, hospitalization, eye problems, nerve damage, the greater risk of infection, heart and organ failure, and even amputation. They know all the likely drugs that a diabetic will need over a year, and so with extraordinary precision they can predict what it will cost to cover that patient. It doesn't matter to them at all whether that figure is $500 a month or $1000 a month, because like the drug company, they're simply going to mark up the cost to cover their overhead and generate a profit for their shareholders. (In the old days, most insurance companies were "mutual" companies, meaning they were owned by their shareholders, kind of like a co-op is operated for the benefit of members. They were less interested in generating a profit since that causes higher prices that would have only been paid by the members anyway, but today most insurance companies are publicly traded, meaning their sole motivation is profits.)

As we saw with the drug companies, insurers are happy to have a more expensive plan because a 30 percent markup on $1000 a month drops $300 to the bottom line as opposed to $150 with a policy that is half as expensive. Multiply that by say, a million premium payers, and it yields an astonishing $3.6 billion in annual profits, compared to only $1.8 billion. Which company would you rather work for, one that makes nearly $4 billion a year or one that nets less than half that? Which one would you rather invest in? You see how it works now and why there is no motivation to have a lower drug cost.

Perhaps you're wondering though, since the consumer ends up paying the premium, why doesn't he reject this higher pricing model? Well, the first reason is one we've already alluded to; John and Jane Doe, with their college degrees and nice house and two new cars and their 2.4 children (well, it's more like 1.4 now), and their regular vacations, spoil themselves at every opportunity, and they're certainly not going to cut corners when it comes to their health, so if given the option between the Chevy coverage or the Cadillac coverage, they choose the Cadillac coverage almost all the time. They might even justify it by saying that yes, there is a small gain, but if that gain makes up the difference—either between life and death or even a more enjoyable life, or one free of pain—then that is worth any cost. In fact, our whole culture is pretty much based on this concept, isn't it? We'll pay anything (in blood, sweat, tears, or personal agony) to get more of something or to avoid pain.

The second reason why the consumer doesn't care is because he doesn't really feel the pain of paying that premium. Most Americans have insurance that is paid for by someone else, namely, their employer. Sure, that employer is paying for the insurance out of money that otherwise would have gone straight to the employee, but since the employee never really had the money in

Off the Grid with Diabetes

his hand and didn't have to write that huge check, he doesn't feel the brunt of that cost. It's a lot like his taxes; most citizens would be outraged at the level of taxation if they had to write a different check each month to all the state and federal agencies to pay all the different taxes (that usually add up to 50 percent of a person's income), but because those taxes are withheld and the employer takes care of it automatically, they don't feel it. They look at the net paycheck, the amount they live on and the amount they've become accustomed to since their very first job in high school, and so the pain is largely avoided. See a trend here?

If you're thinking that your doctor may be the last line of defense against higher or unnecessary drug costs, think again. Your doc has no financial incentive to prescribe lower cost drugs. In fact, it's quite the opposite. In most cases, your doctor doesn't have a direct financial interest in whether or not you use a high cost drug or not. (Although this is changing quickly though as doctors are increasingly forming groups that have a profit interest in insurers or drug companies.) However, what doctors do have an incentive to do is see you frequently, enabling them to bill the insurer more often, to perform more expensive and complex tests, especially if they are the latest and greatest in technology (since this helps to protect them from liability suits, lest something is missed in their diagnosis), and of course, they want to be available to sell you the Cadillac treatment plan. Who wants to sell stripped down Chevys when you can sell the top of the line Cadillac, and after all, the consumer certainly doesn't care if it costs more.

Worse, every party involved also has an interest in the latest and greatest drugs. The pharmaceutical company, after investing tens of millions of dollars in research and development, gets a patent on that drug and wants to sell as much of it as possible before that patent expires in ten years (and the generic version floods the market, driving the price down and making it less profitable).

So the pharmaceutical company is constantly engaged in a planned obsolescence campaign. Planned obsolescence is usually a term that refers to products that are designed to fail after a certain time, requiring a new purchase. Well, as much as drug companies complain about losing patent protection after only ten years of government-protected monopoly, they are secretly thrilled because they will continue to make money forever on the generic versions while having the incentive to roll out a new, better, and of course, more expensive version of the drug.

When a patent expires, a company rarely fails to capitalize on this opportunity by introducing a new upgraded version of the drug. Perhaps it works a little better (at much increased prices), or maybe it has fewer side effects (also at greatly increased costs). Either way, if it is sufficiently different to merit a new patent, they've just gained another ten years of government-protected monopoly. Think about the economics: over the course of ten years, a drug price will have doubled at least once, possibly as much as twice, as inflation has driven the retail price up.

However, herbal and all natural treatments aren't able to be patented, creating two problems. First, if there is no patent, then there is no monopoly, and competition will drive the price down, depressing profits. Secondly, if the treatment is all-natural and doesn't require an expensive laboratory and lots of lobbyists and federal approval, then any old "Joe" can acquire the product, perhaps even grow it in his backyard garden, and the opportunity to gain a dominant, profitable position in the marketplace is greatly reduced.

The insurance company and doctor are similarly threatened by natural and alternative treatments. Why go to a doctor who must bill the insurance company to make your visit economically viable if you could use the Internet to look up the natural ingredients for an herbal solution to your illness? How would an insurance company justify charging you $1000 a month in premiums if your chronic disease and suffering could be alleviated by natural

Off the Grid with Diabetes

products you could buy at a farmer's market, grocery store, or even grow in your survival garden next to the tomatoes?

Thus, the entire pharmaceutical industry, as well as the medical practitioners and government regulators, are opposed to natural or alternative treatments. There's no money to be made distributing them, regulating them, insuring them, or prescribing them. Or rather, there's not nearly as much money to be made, since clearly there are some companies in the natural and alternative medicine business. If you don't believe me, after you've finished with this book, take a few ideas to your local physician and say, "I'm thinking of trying _____ in place of the drug you're currently prescribing; what do you think?" I'm virtually certain he'll have all sorts of reasons why not to, the least of which will be that you might die! He can't bill an insurance company or collect co-pays from a dead person, after all!

This overview ignores an even more important question than evaluating the motives of the various parties—whether or not the drugs they are pushing on us are effective and safe.

The technological advances of the last twenty years have been extraordinary, and it is undeniable that a great many drugs have been developed that are managing disease and pain and prolonging life. However, at the same time, think about those warnings that your pharmacist gives you before administering the prescription, or those awful commercials that take sixty seconds to list the side effects: swelling, trouble breathing, dizziness, headache, fatigue, rapid heartbeat, impotence, hot flashes, sweating, liver failure, heart failure, even death! These are common side effects, not rare ones! This epidemic of side effects begs the question of whether or not it is possible to treat diseases without these costly side effects, and whether the drugs are doing damage internally in the hope of treating the disease.

Most of the medications sold in the United States that are designed to treat diabetes are intended to be accompanied by diet and exercise, which de facto also means that the drug isn't intended for people to consume who don't engage in diet and exercise. Of course, in our society of instant gratification, where we live on credit and debt and work second jobs to afford more stuff, we don't want to cure our disease; we want to manage it.

In fact, the entire medical industry is built around management of disease rather than cure or reversal. It is a relatively easy thing for a doctor to prescribe a medication that will reduce your glucose count. You're happy about the lower number, your doctor is happy about the lower number, your pharmacist is happy to be selling you monthly prescriptions, the insurance company is happy that your diabetes is managed, and, naturally, the drug company is happy to have a new customer. But is your body happy with that new chemical in the system? And will you, now that you have a magic pill to take to manage your blood sugar, have the incentive to correct the behavior that led to the diagnosis? In most cases, we can answer "no" to both questions. Your body isn't happy about the foreign chemicals, and you're not likely to fix your lifestyle if you can just take a pill in the morning, or two pills a day, or three pills a day.... or a few pills plus a shot a day, or two shots a day. (You get the point, right?)

Once your body becomes accustomed to a cocktail of drugs, it does its best to adjust to them. Once acclimated, the diagnosis that was once treated suddenly reappears, usually in the form of high blood sugar again, despite the medicine, and the doctor prescribes an increased dosage. This process may happen over and over again until the point where increased dosages still aren't doing it, so an additional drug is added to the mix. In the end, you may end up so confusing your body that it loses all natural ability to heal or grow, and now you find yourself completely dependent on drugs, where any disruption could prove fatal.

As your body is struggling to adjust to the new or changing medicine, pancreatic function is often disrupted and hypoglycemia is the result. Drug-induced hypoglycemia is one of the

---

Off the Grid with Diabetes

most common side effects of insulin and oral medication and one of the most dangerous. Some of the risk factors are consuming more than one type of medication (whether they are both related to blood sugar or not), vigorous exercise (often something that happens when people first get diagnosed and try to find a quick cure), severe dieting or fasting (again, trying to drop weight quickly), the combination of prescription medicine with herbal treatments, and those with existing digestive problems, kidney damage, or heart trouble.

A common problem with medical treatment of diabetes is that the medicine often times cures one problem by "borrowing from Peter to pay Paul." These drugs often times draw upon the nutrients in your body to work. The consequence is nutrient depletion, which can lead to a cascading problem including sickness, general unhealthiness, organ failure, and even other immune-related diseases. What happens next? You guessed it: these symptoms bring about either a change in medication (which starts the cycle all over again and puts further stress on the body) or the combination of drugs greatly complicates the artificial cocktail your body is dealing with. While these drugs may bring your blood sugar down, they rarely reverse the damage done to your organs, particularly the pancreas, and often contribute to their deterioration in fact.

As organ failure progresses, dangerous chemicals in the form of free radicals are generated throughout your body and naturally congregate in the organs designed to deal with these kinds of toxins, such as the pancreas. The organs that struggle with the influx of the chemicals, now further burdened by an attack of free radicals (and possibly already weakened by the high level of sugar in the blood) become inflamed.

The consequence of this domino effect is often loss of eyesight, loss of limbs, and eventually death. The road to that end may be long, as the body is kept alive by an increasing dosage and complexity of medicine, or the end may come suddenly and without warning. Because diabetes and the current treatment is a relatively new phenomenon (as measured against the evolution of our bodies and the speed at which they adapt), science lacks a long-term evaluation of the common treatment methods.

In short, popular treatment methods don't really address the cause of the disease; rather, they treat the symptoms! This is why some professionals call popular blood sugar treatments "band-aid drugs" because they just cover up the symptoms while the underlying problem remains and, in many cases, worsens.

If your physician prescribes a drug to lower your blood sugar and your levels respond, you think you're getting well. If you stop taking the drug, you discover that you are in fact not getting well. Frequently your condition is even worse than before, because organ damage has continued and chemicals are impairing natural processes, or worse, aggravating the disease. Additionally, most people, when seeing the dramatic drop in blood sugar levels following prescription, won't alter their lives. The consequences are enormous.

Sometimes the drugs themselves are more dangerous than the disease they seek to treat. One recent example is Avandia, a widely popular drug that has been linked to heart failure. Avandia and a related drug also appear to greatly increase a woman's risk of bone fracture. Despite the enormous cost of research and development and the extensive testing required before gaining FDA approval, these drugs still made it to market, and it wasn't until morgues started filling up with patients that the drugs were pulled from the market.

Fortunately, the Internet is a wonderful tool to investigate drugs and their side effects. It may be that consumers are already reporting dangerous problems or consequences of drug interaction long before the manufacturer or the FDA has enough data to demand a recall.

Off the Grid with Diabetes

Even more disturbing is the recent evidence which seems to indicate that not only can we not cure diabetes through chemical treatment, but that toxic chemicals in our body (from medicine or antibiotics) may actually bring on diabetes. One example is prednisone, a cortisone treatment that can damage the pancreas, which we already know is central to insulin production and regulation.

Antibiotics may also be a culprit, because their frequent or prolonged use can destroy the internal flora that is responsible for managing fungi level. Without the natural flora to control fungal growth, fungal infections can arise, leading to further metabolic disorders, ultimately leading to high blood sugar levels. This was first reported by **Family Practice News** in the December 15, 2004, issue.

More concerning is the evidence that artificial insulin is itself toxic. In fact, fatal reactions to insulin are not unheard of. Humulin, which is a common form of manufactured insulin, is genetically engineered and contains contaminants that can lead to allergic shock.

Because Type 1 diabetes is seen by most medical professionals as a "hopeless" disease (meaning we can't cure it), there's a certain amount of apathy about treatment. This can be summed up by the common treatment: prescribe increasing amounts of insulin until the patient dies. But the underlying cause of the disease, largely suspected to be massive toxicity accompanied by fungal infection, is left untreated.

At the same time, one source of Type 1 diabetes seems to be a virus that targets the pancreas. Mention this to your physician, and he is likely to laugh and mock the suggestion, but the data is incontrovertible. After a major viral epidemic, the frequency of Type 1 diabetes often increases exponentially. That is not to say that the viral breakout itself causes the pancreatic damage that leads to Type 1 diabetes (although this is certainly plausible); rather the latest thinking is that widespread use of contaminated vaccines may introduce altered viruses that the body is not familiar with, which in turn infect the organs such as the liver and pancreas. **The Journal of Pediatric Endocrinology** documented a 30 percent increase in the risk of Type 1 diabetes in the vaccinated population.

As we have previously discussed, the presence of antibiotics in cow's milk that are designed to treat infection in cows may also be a contributing factor, as are the harsh chemicals used in the production of processed foods, particularly wheat and refined sugar. Imagine using harsh chemicals to clean your kitchen, getting some of it on your food, and then consuming it; if you became sick immediately afterwards, you might suspect a link!

Before we wrap up this chapter, I want to say a few things about one of the leading public voices on diabetes. The standard diet recommended by the American Diabetes Association relies largely on constant snacking throughout the day as a way of maintaining a steady level of blood sugar. The idea of course is to avoid a massive spike in your blood sugar and the resulting surge of insulin if you eat a big meal only a few times a day. If you don't snack, then your adrenal glands can get tired, and good hormones, such as DHEA, drop, which can cause the insulin resistance to aggravate. Snacking helps diabetics who have trouble storing glycogen too and can prevent hypoglycemia.

However, like the mainstream medical profession, the ADA seems consumed merely with managing the level rather than treating the disease or reversing it. Snacking can cause a lot of problems for people who are relatively newly diagnosed with diabetes, because in the presence of already high insulin levels, snacking will do more damage than good.

Remember that in a healthy person, insulin levels rise after eating to aid in digestion and then after a few hours return to normal. The pancreas goes into a relative rest mode and makes

Off the Grid with Diabetes

glucagon, which tells your liver to release sugar in order to maintain a stable supply in your blood. This is how your body maintains a natural level of stable blood sugar.

When this process begins, your body knows to go looking for a snack—not from the outside, but from the inside in the form of fat! In particular, the body loves to burn triglycerides at this time. But if you snack all day, you preempt the body's normal process. Your eating causes the release of insulin, which means the trigger that is caused by your pancreas' resting never happens. That in turn means that the liver never gets to do its job and triglycerides build up rather than being burned off!

When this happens, as it so often does with diabetics, triglycerides begin to flood your system, and when the physician sees the counts, he prescribes a cholesterol treatment that is often a statin drug. These statins depress your cholesterol numbers into the normal range, but they don't reverse the damage that is done, nor do they attempt to trigger the normal, natural, and healthy way of dealing with triglycerides. It's kind of like the drunk who drinks a lot of coffee while he's getting drunk, thinking that by boosting his metabolism he can burn off all that alcohol he's taking in. The smart thing to do is to just stop drinking and let the body heal itself!

But the ADA, your physician, and the whole healthcare structure are happy with you on diabetic medicine and cholesterol-lowering drugs. Everyone is getting paid, your numbers—for the time being—are in control, and you're seeing results without making significant changes. In reality, your body is in turmoil, your organs are wearing out, and you're getting sicker by the day.

In reality, fat isn't really the problem. Fat is slow to digest and fails to elicit a significant insulin response. Further, foods high in fat are often dense sources of nutrients that naturally combat diabetes. Good examples of this would be red meat, poultry, fatty fish and eggs, staples of diets among natives like the Inuit who experience very low incidents of diabetes in their natural state. These nutrients include thiamine, niacin, pyridoxine, biotin inositol, choline, pantothenic acid, folic acid, vitamin B12, zinc, copper, and magnesium. They are all nutrients known to be anti-diabetic, or more positively, pro-life. Zinc in particular is essential for the creation of natural insulin and is found in rich amounts in red meat, poultry, and fatty fish, all now blacklisted on most Western menus because fat is supposedly bad for you. Obviously the organic, natural products are the ones we're speaking of here, because the commercially raised livestock we are accustomed to eating have been fed an unnatural cocktail designed to pump up weight at the expense of the nutritional value and will be full of drugs which have no place in your system.

In conclusion, the entire health care system, from the point of service through the drug manufacturer, and even our modern Western gratification-based society encourages destructive and expensive behavior. It bears an uncanny similarity to the economic crisis which has devastated our economy in recent years; politicians in Congress wanted to encourage homeownership for their own political benefit, so they created federal subsidy programs in the form of Fannie and Freddie, the FHA, VA, and insurance programs. Banks saw these as guarantees and so were more eager to lend where they otherwise never would have. Brokers borrowed that money and lent to everyone with a pulse, and borrowers who could never get a loan before gobbled them up eagerly. Those loans were bundled into securities that agencies—paid to rate them positively—guaranteed were risk free, and everyone from pension funds to banks to governments bought all they could get, seeing a high-yield, risk-free investment. When it collapsed, the dominos cascaded across the world. The system was designed, perhaps unintentionally, to fail. The same is the case with modern medicine, except this is your life, and you can change things. Let's find out how!

Off the Grid with Diabetes

Chapter Four:

External Threats to Your Health

If you are reading this book, the odds are you're already concerned about risks that may alter our modern lifestyles in dramatic and adverse ways. In this chapter, we'll review some of those potential disruptions and explore the possible consequences and whether those consequences will impact your life.

Our modern society is an extremely delicate one. With the advancements in our technology and their proliferation throughout society, life has taken on a new reliance on technology that no generation before has ever lived with. This reliance on technology has reached dependency levels. Few Americans exist without a day-to-day reliance on some aspect of technology to maintain their standard of living.

The electricity we require to maintain our homes, businesses, and entertainment is increasingly produced by a few centrally located power sources and is increasingly stretched to cover an ever-growing consumption brought on by more personal and business devices. Our water supply is increasingly dependent on the treatment of wastewater as our fresh water sources grow more rare and precious. Without the centralized, expensive, and complex chemical treatments, many of our communities would have no reliable source of potable water. Our methods of communication, whether they are cell phones, Internet, email, voice over IP services (which now provide most long distance and Internet based calls, such as Skype), and of course Wi-Fi, all utilize technology that originated in the last generation and have been so quickly updated or replaced that devices built just five years ago are often incompatible.

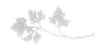 # Off the Grid with Diabetes

With this advancement in technology comes an increasing requirement that devices operate with precision and predictability across a range of systems. The slightest disruption at any link in the chain can lead to a failure, and yet, life is increasingly dependent on these kinds of transactions. If during a voice call there is a problem, you may hear an echo, static, disruption, a delay or even a dropped call: we all know how irritating that is. Furthermore, when the system is put under stress, it can collapse. Those who have lived through natural disasters, terrorist acts, or even just localized breaking news events know that usage can spike and overload the system, leading to busy signals or the inability to access a network, to place or receive calls, and even to access 911.

Our businesses, and certainly the health care profession, are dependent upon these systems for maintaining the level of care to which we've become accustomed. Understanding the fragility of the network helps to recognize how easily things can be disrupted. It doesn't require an "end of the world" type event for our lives to experience dramatic change.

Additionally, we are currently experiencing a rate of change that is very high relative to what previous generations of our ancestors experienced. A man now in his 80s has seen the world change in ways that were unforeseen by his parents: a world in which manned flight has gone from a dream to a common unremarkable reality experienced by millions daily. He has lived through a revolution in which the majority of mankind has gone from candlelight to mobile, cheap electricity and from outdoor latrines to efficient, safe, and clean indoor plumbing. That same man's life expectancy has gone from 60 to 85, an increase of nearly 50 percent!

Early in his life, that man would have known of the telegraph, and now he has virtually free access to live video conferencing with anyone in the world. Billions of people now have regular access to a physician; in a previous generation, those same people would have lived an entire lifetime having never seen a doctor.

Off the Grid with Diabetes

Our health care system is as fragile as any. With the rapidity of technological development, infrastructure fragility increases at a rate even faster than 1:1. By that I mean that when we introduce something new and unfamiliar, or even unproven, there are glitches that sometimes make us wonder if the development really represents progress. Remember how you first experimented with computers, and how things seemed so awkward and frustrating, and how the computer would lock up and crash, occasionally shut down, or delete data? Ever have an experience with a corrupted hard drive or operating system or a virus? Weeks, months, even years of data can be lost. And yet, as we grow more comfortable with the systems, we never think about going back to the typewriter and carbon copies.

Our health care system is at this same kind of juncture and is undergoing true revolutionary changes. The fragility of the system has increased dramatically. Things are more centralized than ever. Providers at every level of the system are more integrated and interdependent than ever before, and even at the

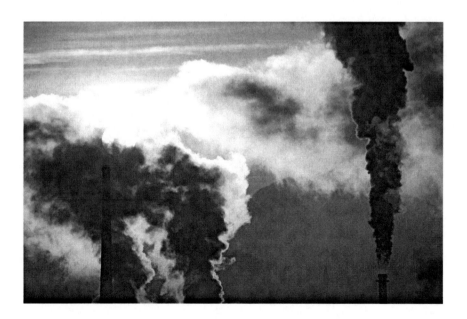

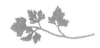

point of service, individual employees cannot perform their duties unless they are integrated in real time with data that may be stored on a computer located in India or China. Even something as simple as setting an appointment or making a copy of your insurance card might prove to be impossible if there's a glitch on a network computer 5,000 miles away!

It doesn't take an event of great significance for our lives to be disrupted. Something as simple as a computer virus may wipe out your prescription at the pharmacy, leaving them unable to access your account, verify your insurance coverage, or even determine what medication is on hand! A tornado effecting one suburb in the Deep South may take a network link off line that prevents your doctor from accessing his patient database, leaving him unable to review your past records (this actually happened to a large portion of the medical community following the tornadoes that destroyed Joplin, Missouri).

An event need not be catastrophic to affect our lives. Simply touching a critical pressure point upon which many other processes rely can cause chaos. And of course if an event is catastrophic, regardless of how rare, the effects will far-reaching and disastrous. Getting struck by lightning is highly unlikely, but if it does occur, it has a serious impact on your life.

These events are sometimes called "Black Swan" events. They are extremely rare, but when they happen, they bring about so much change (and sometimes chaos), that their importance cannot be underestimated. Because these events are often times so disruptive, we have a tendency to try to ignore them. We don't like to think about such unpleasantness, let alone plan for it. And yet, these are the very things to which we should give the most attention.

The Richter scale by which earthquakes are measured is a great prism through which to view these events. Events which measure low on the scale are more common and of lower intensity. As you

Off the Grid with Diabetes

move higher up the scale, the frequency diminishes substantially, but the power, intensity, and ultimate devastation are hundreds of times greater!

The same is true with the risks that present threats to our lifestyle. There are many more hurricanes, tornados, and blizzards than there are asteroids that impact the earth causing extinction events, and yet, if the asteroid does hit, the consequences will be far-reaching and more deadly than a tsunami off the coast of Japan, and look at how deadly that isolated event was for the people in its path!

In our everyday life, we face many risks that we cannot avoid but which we try to mitigate. We hope they won't happen, but in recognition that we can't guarantee against their occurrence and keeping in mind the possible consequences, we seek to offset that risk or spread it around. We do this through insurance.

In the unlikely event something bad happens, we want to have built up a hedge of sorts to help mitigate that risk. In our lives we may not expect to ever need brain surgery, but we want to have a health insurance policy that would cover the high six-figure expense if it does happen. A stay-at-home mother may not expect her thirty-year-old husband to die tomorrow, but if he does, she wants to have life insurance that will help offset the loss of his income, so she and the young children are not homeless and reduced to handouts.

When we acquire insurance, we are forgoing the use of those dollars today for the benefit they will give us in the event of that catastrophic event. There is, of course, the possibility that catastrophe will not happen. In fact, we hope it doesn't happen, but we are hedging against its possibility. I'm sharing this insurance analogy because it is central to our philosophy of preparing for an off-grid potentiality.

I don't want something terrible to happen, but it's possible. There's a lot about our modern society that I don't like, but I sure

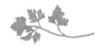

wish there was a way to correct those things gently without a world-altering event. It would be nice if a gentle correction could bring us back into precise balance and alignment, but history suggests otherwise. We know that in Noah's time the world required an adjustment, and it was rapid, dramatic, involved catastrophic human loss and suffering, and led to the rebirth of the world.

We can't know what the future holds, but we can study the past to learn what is possible and study it to learn how we can prepare for ourselves and our descendants. Many so-called survivalists or preppers respond to this call by stockpiling food and weapons in their homes, and this is a good first step, but not the last. Eventually, that food will run out; the key for long-term survival is knowledge and relationships.

Man is not a solitary animal, but a social being. God did not create Adam alone in the garden to hoard his food, but gave him Eve and called them to cultivate the garden together. We too must consider that as humans we thrive in communities, not hiding away in caves or underground bunkers. For our best and highest purposes, we require multiple skills, diverse experiences, and many components to weather the storms that bring about illness, injury, and death in our lives. We cannot ignore the social aspects either; studies have found that people who live in solitary conditions for long periods frequently develop mental illness and often regress into animal-like conditions.

The likelihood of any event undoing thousands of years of technological advancement, bringing about a cave-man-type existence seems to me to be very unlikely. Regardless of the severity, any remnant will possess the vast accumulation of discovery, knowledge, and experience possessed by the human race at the present time. It won't be forgotten altogether. Human beings also have the proven ability to rebound from even the most catastrophic events. We need to remember the complete devastation of Europe and Japan after World War II, where entire cities

Off the Grid with Diabetes

had been wiped off the face of the earth, and see how they have been repopulated and rebuilt. The lessons we learn from these experiences remind us that the wide dispersal of knowledge is critical, as is the mobility of man (we cannot pretend that we can live tied to one location when circumstances may make that impossible), and those with emotional and spiritual preparation do the best during times of recovery and quickly rise in positions of leadership and influence.

These last two characteristics—spiritual and emotional preparations—cannot be underestimated. Those who have considered these possibilities, accepted that they may be inevitable, and recognized that they are part of God's plan, leading to good regardless of the suffering, can adjust more quickly, recognizing in them the opportunity to rebuild, to serve those who are needy, to heal the sick, or to teach and lead the ignorant.

In this chapter we will review many threats to our lifestyle, but the list is by no means a comprehensive review of every imaginable catastrophe. You may think that some important possibilities have been omitted or that those included are absurd, but the objective is to brainstorm the possibilities so you can evaluate your "insurance" options. Clearly some threats are more likely than others. Some may be more relevant to you, e.g., a hurricane is a more relevant threat if you live near the coast, while an epidemic may be a greater risk if you live in an urban area with a great deal of immigration or foreign inbound travelers. Some risks are remote, but may have such potential life-changing consequences that they cannot be ignored. The possibility of solar flares that may disable our communications systems or damage our electrical grid, leaving it off line for years, might fall into this category.

It's not hard to imagine a scenario where your employer might eliminate your health care coverage. If health insurance premiums continue to rise at rates approaching 25 percent a year, if a small group policy experiences substantial losses and

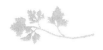

coverage is difficult to acquire, if the business is losing money or goes out of business altogether, if a new owner chooses to end or restrict benefits, or if you lose your job, you may suddenly find yourself without affordable, reliable coverage.

Nor is it difficult to envision a scenario where you are not eligible for coverage. Like many millions of Americans who are under-employed, you may have part-time or independent contractor work that does not provide for health benefits. And yet, unless you are young, old, or very sick, government aid programs may not cover you. This is presently the case with tens of millions of Americans.

At the same time, we are seeing the nationalization of our private health plan through Obamacare, which threatens states' rights, our individual liberties (as a result of the individual mandate), the private health care system itself, and the market's confidence in our commitment to the free market. Further, the administration has made no qualms about pursuing a system that would emulate that of England or Canada.

We know from experience that although everyone in those nations technically has access to health care at little or no cost, the population experiences rationing, long delays, lower quality of service, and the predictable loss of quality that comes under any Marxist program. Our own nation is host to the wealthy from these nations who can afford to travel and hire the best medical coverage available. Where will Americans go in the future for their health care, and will you be among the elite who can afford it?

We can learn what happens when a plan of nationalization is put in place, thanks to the experiments across Europe and here in the U.S. in the twentieth century. One of the first market responses is the increase in prices. It's a simple economic rule: if supply is fixed and demand suddenly rises, prices will rise. If, as Obama hopes, all Americans are forced to buy health insurance (those policies approved by the government), then prices for the

Off the Grid with Diabetes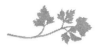

same coverage will rise in relation to what they were the day before. If tens of millions of people are suddenly forced into the system, there is no possible way there can be an immediate, corresponding increase in the supply of doctors, nurses, skilled assistants, supplies, or even drugs. These things can adjust in time and undoubtedly many entrepreneurs will rush to fill the gap between supply and demand, but in the interim, consumers will see higher prices, longer wait times, shortages, and a reduced level of care.

As prices skyrocket and services become scarce, the government will want to shield itself from responsibility and seek to manage prices, falling back on blaming speculators and accusing doctors, hospitals, pharmacists, and insurers of price gouging. Sound familiar? The same approach has been taken with other industries where government intrusion led to shortages and the predictable and corresponding rise in prices.

When prices rise rapidly, it's called hyperinflation. Setting aside the possibility of a health crisis helping to feed hyperinflation, our nation's current economic policy, combined with the monetary policy of the Fed, makes this a very real possibility.

As inflation creeps up, it becomes difficult for businesses to make money, so they do their best to get rid of dollars quickly by buying things of tangible value, be that land, buildings, natural resources, inventory they can sell, or liquid assets that are not denominated in American dollars (such as stocks in the Euro Zone, Canadian dollars, Australian dollars, or even Swiss Francs). Of course, the rich already do this because a) they can and b) they have access to the best financial and legal advice and know the likelihood of hyperinflation given our history.

As businesses and the wealthy try to get rid of the dollar, the pace of its loss in value hastens. That causes further loss in confidence. When no one wants something, it becomes difficult to trade that thing for something of actual value. As the federal

---

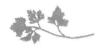

Off the Grid with Diabetes

government continues to print money by the trillions, these dollars lose value, and foreign investors don't want them either. If that happens quickly, then the Treasury won't be able to borrow enough money to legally finance the Fed's printing of dollars. That could really cause a collapse in the dollar, meaning an overnight devaluation rather than a more traditional long, painful slide. Suddenly you wake up one day and prices have doubled.

How would it impact you if you went to the pharmacist tomorrow and prices had doubled, tripled, or gone up by ten times? It has happened in the modern world, in developed economies. Germany in the 1920s is the prime example, but 100 years ago Argentina was a first-world country with a standard of living higher than that of the U.S. They have lagged behind us ever since their own default and devaluation.

It is not at all inconceivable that our economic problems could put such pressure on the value of the dollar that even here in the United States people would not accept them for commerce, preferring to trade in things of actual value. After all, if you don't want it, why would your doctor or pharmacist? Many people respond to this possibility by saying, "Well, if something like that ever did happen, 'they' would fix it". This mysterious "they" refers to the same people who got us into this mess, the same people who believe more borrowing and leverage is the way out of a crisis brought on by too much borrowing and leverage.

Because we as a nation have such a spectacular history of overcoming challenges and recovering more quickly than our cousins across the pond, we've become delusional about how we could respond to such a crisis. To look in the rear view mirror as a roadmap for the future is dangerous; in fact, it is because we have abandoned the recipe for success that gave us so many victories in the past that the future now looks so bad, and a generation of leaders weaned on poisoned milk is unlikely to suddenly develop a taste for what is healthy when they have never tasted it in the first place.

Off the Grid with Diabetes

Wishing therefore for a quick solution to our current problem or a fast recovery from a collapse, is dangerous. If and when a hyper-inflationary scenario becomes real, it is likely to last for months, perhaps even years. The book **Atlas Shrugged** by Ayn Rand is popular in large part because it so accurately depicts how a formerly free nation slides into a period of economic stagnation and deterioration. The crisis doesn't develop overnight, and the resolution doesn't come quickly. Worse, as long as both doctors and the patient are in denial about the real problem, an adequate treatment plan cannot be devised, let alone embarked upon.

Therefore it seems likely that when economic cracks in our foundation do bring about hiccups in our health care system, it is likely that they will persist for some time. Medical professionals will slowly start leaving the field, entering into private, cash practices, or retiring earlier to pursue other endeavors that are not so highly regulated. Drug companies, finding no one able to pay for their expensive medications, will stop making them. Insurers will not want to accept dollars from you today for coverage of a year's worth of expenses if prices are rising at the rate of

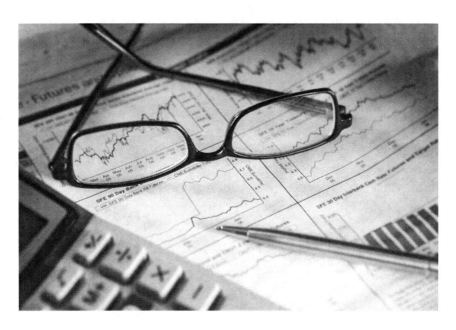

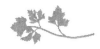
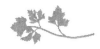

10, 20, 50, or 100 percent a year. Their objective is to invest your premiums and make money, not lose it the first day your check clears! At the same time, pharmacists will quickly go out of business, with no products to sell and no customers to buy them anyway.

Think it can't happen here? Who would have imagined just twenty years ago that we would be having the debate we are today? Who would have imagined that most of the ten planks of the Communist Manifesto would have been implemented to one degree or another in our country? Who would have imagined that tax rates are on average ten times higher than what the highest rate was when the federal income tax was instituted in the 1920s? Who would have dreamed that the federal government would consume more than 20 percent of the total economy, and that combined tax rates would average 50 percent of income (considering federal tax, Medicare, Medicaid, social security, state and local income tax, and state and local sales taxes)?

How long will it take before men who espouse political views contrary to that of the administration are imprisoned? In fact, it is already happening. A man in Chicago was charged with a federal crime for urging the people to use jury nullification as a check on the abuse of power by federal judges. In this environment, if a man can go to prison for urging lawful, nonviolent legal resistance to tyranny, how long will it be before some classes of people are placed at the back of the line for access to health care? If you can be put in prison for expressing yourself, what is it to deny you health care? Prison requires a judicial accomplice, but your health care could be suspended by executive action, since it is executive agencies that regulate Obamacare.

Inasmuch as some conservative activists have already been characterized as potential domestic terrorists (tea party attendees, tax protesters, pro-lifers, and second amendment defenders), how much of a stretch would it be to deny health care to so-called "enemies of the state"?

Off the Grid with Diabetes

This political environment is precisely what has led so many governments around the world to succumb to a revolutionary Marxist leadership. Throughout Latin America, Europe, Russia, and China, radical activists have infiltrated the courts, tax agencies, legislative branches, and the military to facilitate the proper interpretation and implementation of agendas in alignment with their precepts. The final step involves the control of law enforcement, education, and health care, both to reward the supplicants and punish those who resist.

Already some medical professionals are under attack for not bowing to government dictates. Catholic Charities, one of the largest health care providers in the U.S. and one of the biggest employers in the industry, is having to consider whether to comply with federal requirements that it provide abortions and support adoptions by homosexual couples, or to simply close its doors, ending services to millions, particularly the needy. Similar pressure is being brought to bear on hospitals and pharmacists who do not want to prescribe morning-after abortion pills.

Most medical professionals are dependent on the government for a large portion of their revenue. Federal agencies, through Medicare, Medicaid, Social Security, Disability, or the Veterans Administration, make possible the large overhead that doctors require to see the large numbers of patients they're responsible for. Just imagine the consequences if even a few doctors or provider networks were to exit, finding their religious convictions at odds with legal requirements.

But our health care is not at risk just from nefarious agents in government and among the left. An epidemic of natural or terrorist origins can easily bring our system to its knees. The common experience at a physician's office during flu season or when the cable news networks report a possible outbreak of some rare but deadly disease can remind us of the first stages of a true epidemic. The long lines, difficulty getting an appointment, little to no time with a physician, and hurried and rude staff short of sleep

and overwhelmed is hardly a pleasant or effective experience. You might even have trouble getting through to the receptionist as phone lines become overwhelmed as every person with a cough or sniffle calls in to their doctor asking for an over-the-phone diagnosis, or an in-person assurance. Think I'm overstating the fact? Do we as a nation not demand—as some sort of birthright—the very best of everything? Do we not run out to the stores and clean the shelves of every "necessity" at the first sign of inclement weather?

If and when a real epidemic does hit, many of the first casualties will be medical professionals and first responders. Once ill, these professionals will either exit the work force altogether or have greatly reduced efficiency, further compounding the problem. Your physician, if a typical family practitioner, may manage 2,000 patients. If that one physician is ill, the lives of a huge number of people are affected. Epidemics in past eras, including the black plague in Europe, claimed as much as 30 percent of the population, while inflicting nearly 50 percent losses on medical professionals and those involved in caring for the ill (or transporting bodies).

It's easy to dismiss comparisons with the thirteenth century as irrelevant, but their primary problem was ignorance of the nature (and cause) of the disease. It's not inconceivable that a fast moving contagion would spread more quickly than our medical professionals could identify it and develop a treatment. After all, we still do not have a cure for AIDS, and we have spent many billions of dollars on this relatively minor disease (when compared with heart disease and cancers which claim so many more lives).

When an epidemic does occur, national emergency response plans include a possible quarantine for thirty to ninety days— or whatever is deemed necessary by the national command authority—to allow the disease to kill the sick and then die out while limiting its exposure. The problem is that in comparison to previous generations of men, we travel far more widely, more quickly, and more often. Huge portions of our population travel

Off the Grid with Diabetes

daily, many of them internationally, and when we consider how many more people come into contact with those travelers, but do not travel themselves, then a significant portion of the population could be infected by a chemical, biological, or viral agent introduced into the population.

Some experts have predicted that even with quarantine, 30 percent of the population could die within ninety days.

When you consider that most people are not prepared to last that long in terms of food and water, it raises the question about those who are dependent on their medication for survival. It is one thing to skip meals; it is another to skip medication that may manage your blood sugar or blood pressure or regulate your heart rate. These kinds of threats seem remote, but the odds of an epidemic continue to rise as we regularly travel into more rugged, wild areas of the globe.

While a plague may seem like something out of a movie and easily dismissed as a science fiction fantasy, our collapsing infrastructure is a very real thing. By bipartisan consensus, our national infrastructure needs are in the trillions of dollars.

While arguments rage about what the proper role of the government is in maintaining roads, bridges, dams, and railways, or whether states instead of the federal government should be involved, or whether it should all be a private affair, the deterioration is something no one denies. As our roads, bridges, and utilities begin to wear out, transportation will be affected, both in terms of our travel times and the expense. If bad roads are avoided, longer routes lead to delayed and more expensive transportation, and if the bad roads are not avoided, similar costs are experienced through damages, higher maintenance costs, and delays associated with closures and detours.

We already know that our food comes from hundreds, and in some cases thousands, of miles away, but our sources of medicine are even more centralized in far-flung, highly urban and developed

---

areas. Bridges connect the rest of the country to these narrow corridors where laboratories experiment and manufacture drugs that keep us alive. Of course, pharmacies, hospitals, and doctors' offices are all dependent upon roadways, bridges, and airports to receive their supplies (and for us to reach them!).

As few as three bridges across the Mississippi affect 30 percent of all the interstate movement of merchandise in the U.S., and a failure of any one of these bridges would have an adverse impact on nearly 100 million people in the direct aftermath. Even if your drugs come from a different source, you can be assured of shortages and price increases as the national supply is instantly impacted by a failure or closure of just one key bridge.

Additionally, most big cities in the U.S. rely on bridges as well (since waterways are so key to commerce and agriculture), so even short-distance travel and commutes are easily disrupted by infrastructure problems. Of course, employers are dependent on the mobility of their employees, as are law enforcement agencies.

It's not just the delivery of the drugs though; it's the movement of all of the people to their workplaces. If the doctor lives just a mile from the hospital but can't get there because a bridge is out, it doesn't matter that drugs could be flown in by helicopter. Of course, on a more personal level, if you can't get to your physician because of a road outage, it doesn't matter whether the doctor can or not. If the bridge is out on your side of town and the ambulance can't reach you, then nothing else matters.

Unfortunately, our infrastructure issues aren't limited to just crumbling bridges and roads. Our electrical grid is aging, vulnerable to failure, overload, cyber assault, strategic attack (in the form of electromagnetic pulse), and naturally occurring solar flares.

It has been widely reported that our grid relies on fifty-year-old technology and parts. Many of those components are obsolete and are difficult to replace. The replacements are often

---

Off the Grid with Diabetes

manufactured overseas, and there is a backlog on many of the most critical components, such as transformers. These electrical bottlenecks are fragile and vulnerable to overload as well as terrorist attacks. Current estimates put the actual backlog in orders at two years—meaning an order for new parts today cannot be filled for twenty-four months!

At some point, a smart terrorist will stop planning large, difficult, and expensive attacks on national monuments and high-profile urban areas and begin to attack our weak, unprotected electrical grid. No one guards these vulnerable substations and transformers, and the expertise and equipment needed to damage or disable them is elementary. Imagine a dedicated force of just 100 insurgents roaming the country attacking key points and disrupting our grid. What can be blown up, stolen, or simply damaged beyond repair in a matter of seconds may take weeks, months, or even years to replace.

The threat to the grid is real as well. In fact, cyber assaults on the grid are already suspected and may be the cause of previous regional blackouts that affected tens of millions over the last decade. Cyberterrorists can infiltrate the computers that manage the electrical supply and disrupt normal operations with just a few clicks on the keyboard.

Similarly, our grid is vulnerable to electromagnetic attack from the atmosphere. Any nation or group that can launch an inter-continental missile could detonate a nuclear device high above the country, potentially permanently damaging any complex electrical device over an entire region. Although some basic steps can be taken to protect electrical devices from this kind of pulse weapon, the cost for the entire grid is substantial and so far has not been budgeted for. Even presidential candidate Newt Gingrich has publicly discussed the Congress' research into this question and the urgent need for action.

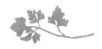 # Off the Grid with Diabetes

The mainstream media has also latched on to the predictions of scientists who have noted a regularly occurring cycle of solar flares and accurately predicted substantial increases in solar activity, which could have a devastating effect on satellites, aircraft, and even ground equipment. In fact, at the time of this writing, international airlines have had their flight plans altered to keep air traffic away from the poles, where the atmosphere offers less protection from the damaging solar activity.

While rerouting of international air traffic may not seem to be much of a concern, the potential for explosive solar activity and the devastating consequences are easy to see. Huge portions of our communications rely on satellite equipment, not to mention the GPS system on which so many consumers and our national defense rely. If only our satellites, beyond the protection of our atmosphere, were damaged, the consequences would be enormous, but if land-based equipment or the thousands of aircraft in the air at any moment around the world were damaged as well, the consequences would be unimaginable.

It's easy to see how our electrical grid could be damaged and how even a short-term existence without electricity would alter life in extreme ways. Imagine no refrigeration of food or medicine. No cash registers operating, no computers to determine what inventory is on hand and what must be ordered. No power to charge cell phone batteries or power computers. No Internet to communicate or conduct business. No payroll systems to pay employees. No physician access to your health records. No manufacturers of drugs, and no one who can deliver them. All this could happen without a terrorist attack, a nuclear meltdown, or a Y2K-like event; one burst of unusually high levels of solar radiation would bring it all down. Even if it could be restored in a matter of weeks or months, what would the costs be in human lives? If the lights didn't come back on for just three months, how would your life be affected?

Off the Grid with Diabetes

In the last ten years, we've all grown more accustomed to the potential for terrorist attacks in our communities, and we've already considered some of the ways that could manifest itself in our health care. While terrorists remain fixated on high profile, strategic assets, our future almost certainly holds a more modern, Israeli-type experience, where suicide bombings and small, independent groups utilize low technology devices and improvisation to undermine public confidence in our domestic security.

This day-to-day constant threat of violence is something the Israelis have grown accustomed to. We regularly hear reports of armed men and women stopping a terrorist attack in Tel Aviv or Jerusalem, because their population is armed, educated and mentally and emotionally prepared to act in an instant. We exist at the opposite end of the spectrum. As agents investigating the TSA have discovered, even trained airport security officials miss a huge number of weapons during screenings and pat-downs. The average American on the street is not in a position to prevent the kind of low-intensity guerrilla warfare that experts believe is part of our future.

If and when attacks on buses, railways, retail locations, schools, hospitals, and first responders do begin to proliferate, how will that impact health care, or for that matter, our society at large? The direct impact seems obvious; Americans will do what they did in the aftermath of 9/11: they'll stay home.

As consumers retreat to their homes, unsure as to when and where the next attack might happen, the economy will contract. Medical professionals, if they're willing to venture outside their homes, won't want to leave the heavily fortified hospitals and offices.

It's easy to see how social unrest might manifest itself in these conditions. With a depressed economy and people staying at home, hunger and opportunity will drive people to riot and loot. Those inclined in this direction don't need much encouragement, as the trial results of Rodney King and Hurricane Katrina have

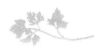

demonstrated. As inventory looting becomes common, businesses will hire law enforcement officers and even soldiers to guard their property. Instead of working in productive capacities, building things of value, our economy will contract further as paranoia grows and we become concerned with protecting life and limb and what little property we may have.

It's easy to predict the effect on your health care universe. Your movement and that of your physician may be limited. There will be shortage of product and higher prices. There may be controls on the currency, and rationing of care is a certainty. Are you prepared to live a healthy life under these circumstances?

We have not even discussed the most likely events to impact your health care—natural disasters. We have significant events happen every day in this world: blizzards, floods, earthquakes, tornados, hurricanes, tsunamis, volcanic eruptions, wildfires, and droughts. That's not including the rare, but catastrophic, asteroid impacts or polar shifts, which can threaten our very existence.

When these catastrophes happen on a local level, they may end life as it is known there, but have little to no impact on people living hundreds of miles away. When they affect a region, the results are more significant. A natural disaster that affects an entire nation sends shock waves around the world.

As the earthquake and ensuing tsunami last year in Japan demonstrated, an event thousands of miles away with no direct influence on us can have far-reaching effects. Financial markets panic, suppliers are disrupted, and food sources come into question as worries about radiation impact our food. Even now epidemiologists are finding increased levels of radiation in our food and milk supplies as a result of the disaster in Japan.

These natural disasters are unpredictable and unavoidable. It's not a question of if, but when. We know they happen. We see them happening all around us. There is very little we can do to

Off the Grid with Diabetes

avoid or mitigate their raw power, although by our choice of living location we can reduce some of their occurrences. But if a solar event brings about a shift of the poles, disrupting all our navigation, communication, and possibly our electrical grid, it doesn't matter whether you live in the mountains of Utah or on an island in the Caribbean, because life will forever be altered.

What will happen if the electricity to our own nuclear power plants is disrupted or the employees stop showing up for work? We have dozens of power plants located around the country, and the event in Japan demonstrates that our experience with failing nuclear power plants is so rudimentary that we cannot accurately predict the potential results of abandonment or failure of power plants. What will the consequences for our environment—our air, water, soil, wild animals, and livestock— and our very existence be if a regional, national, or global event disrupts just our nuclear plant production? It's scary even to contemplate, let alone prepare for.

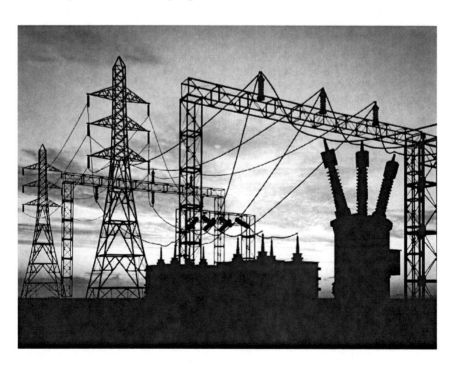

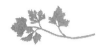

In conclusion, our life is extremely fragile. The sense of normalcy and stability we have is an illusion. The pace of change in our lives is dramatic, but because we are so close and because we have a hard time analyzing what that change means to us, we tend to put the blinders on. For those who have accepted the concept of radical change, preparation is often limited and inadequate. Most of us have done very little in the way of preparing, and for those who have, it tends to be limited to a few MREs in the basement or a few extra jugs of water. These are the kinds of preparations that might help over a long weekend but hardly prepare us to survive and thrive in a real-life disaster.

It's important to stockpile food, supplies, and medicine. You can't expect to last ninety days off the grid without a substantial degree of material possession. If you haven't done a dry run for a weekend and turned the power off to your home and lived for a few days in that condition, you haven't really taken prepping seriously. The stress and emotional pressure (not to mention the anxiety and fear) that will accompany a real disaster are incalculable. Only a solid spiritual foundation can truly prepare you for that.

Your preparation extends far beyond materials you have to stockpile. What you know can never be looted from you. What you know can never be left behind if you are forced to abandon your home or leave your retreat. What you have stockpiled in your mind and heart can be distributed to dozens, hundreds, even thousands of other beneficiaries, just as Christ shared the good news with his twelve apostles, who in turn evangelized the entire world. From those twelve there are now two billion followers.

Over the following chapters I'm going to share with you the good news about the natural and alternative medicinal therapies available to manage, treat, and even reverse the ravages of diabetes without dependence on delivery methods, Big Pharma, Big Government, or even reliable, cheap electricity. Whether you

Off the Grid with Diabetes

have a huge budget and lots of time or just a few dollars, you can take advantage of the miracles God has placed in our food supply and among the weeds at our feet.

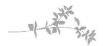
Chapter Five:

Eat Your Way to Health!

If you've read anything about diabetes, it is easy to develop the idea that food is the enemy. In fact, it is true that some foods, namely our modern fast food and processed commercial foods, are the enemy. It's not just the enemy of diabetics, but anyone who is concerned about their long-term health and performance.

Diabetes is a complex metabolic disorder. It is far more complicated than just too much sugar in the diet or blood. The presence of the wrong kinds of sugar in our food (and too much of them) is relevant. Remember, diabetes is more about the way your body deals with sugar and its inability to process it correctly. However, our nation has an addiction to sugar. We eat between 90 to 180 pounds of sugar per person each year. With this in mind, I want to talk a little about sugar, sugar alternatives, and artificial sweeteners.

The overconsumption of sugar and sugar-related additives like high-fructose corn syrup have led to an epidemic of obesity, digestive disorders, autoimmune disorders, thyroid problems, diabetes, the metabolic syndromes (dangerously high cholesterol plus high blood sugar and high blood pressure), and other maladies associated with obesity.

On top of this, our malnourished and over-fed citizenry (that seems like a contradiction, doesn't it?) have the wrong notions about food. The information that I have assembled here is intended to change your attitudes about food and allow you to make informed, unbiased decisions.

In an earlier chapter we spent some time discussing the process that yields refined, processed white sugar and why it is so bad. Yes, it tastes good, looks good, and mixes well in desserts, but it

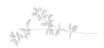

is terrible for you. It suppresses your immune system and human growth hormone production (which help prevent infection) and damages the pancreas. Sugar builds up in your blood and organs and is also stored in the more inactive places in your body, such as your thighs, bottom, and midsection, giving you that spare tire. Stored fat is literally the excess calories you have ingested above and beyond what your body needs.

Your body really is incredible. It recognizes what is excess and wants to keep it on hand in the event that a time comes when there is a shortage of food. Your body will then convert that stored fat—just stored energy—and burn it. Wonderful, right? Well, most of us don't skip too many meals, so that fat never gets burned, and we continue to overeat, storing up more of the fat.

We already know how the pancreas, liver, and kidneys can suffer when they struggle with excess sugar and fat, but your brain is traumatized as well. Scientists have learned that when overwhelmed with sugar and fat, your memory begins to fade, simple math becomes a problem, and you start to have those "senior moments" long before they are justified. The cascade of problems can lead to fatigue, depression, nerve damage, confusion, and a whole variety of other problems that take two, three, or even more combinations of drugs to address.

At the same time, sugar strips your body of many necessary chemicals and minerals. So, when you're purchasing food, one of the first lines of defense is to watch for sugar additives that you may not even realize are in the product. Here are some sugar additives that you might find in the stores that you should keep an eye out for:

Sucrose: A fancy name for the refined, crystallized white sugar

Dextrose: Pure glucose

Lactose: A simple sugar derived from milk

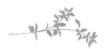

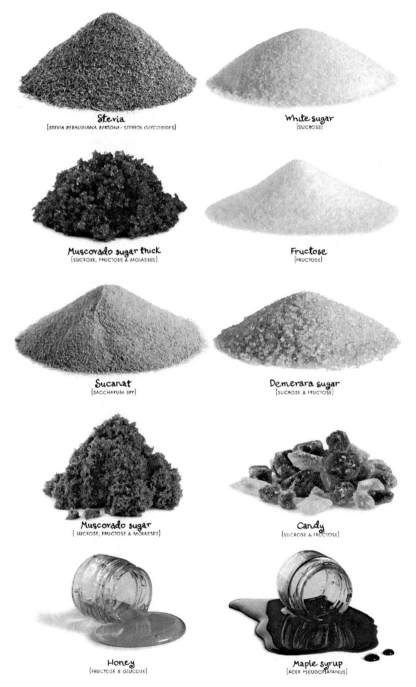

Stevia
[STEVIA REBAUDIANA BERTONI - STEVIOL GLYCOSIDES]

White sugar
[SUCROSE]

Muscovado sugar thick
[SUCROSE, FRUCTOSE & MOLASSES]

Fructose
[FRUCTOSE]

Sucanat
[SACCHARUM SPP]

Demerara sugar
[SUCROSE & FRUCTOSE]

Muscovado sugar
[SUCROSE, FRUCTOSE & MOLASSES]

Candy
[SUCROSE & FRUCTOSE]

Honey
[FRUCTOSE & GLUCOSE]

Maple syrup
[ACER PSEUDOPLATANUS]

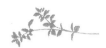

Maltose: A simple sugar derived from grain or starch

Maltodextrin: Manufactured sugar from maltose and dextrose

Brown sugar: Refined sugar coated with molasses or colored with caramel

Raw sugar: White sugar that is not quite as refined with a little molasses remaining

Fructose: A simple sugar made from fruit

Corn syrup: A manufactured syrup made from corn

High fructose corn syrup: A highly concentrated corn syrup

White grape juice: A highly purified fructose solution

Not all of these sugars are equally bad for you. In general, the more processed they are, the worse they are for you, both because the good natural stuff has been removed and because lots of artificial stuff has been added. Let's review some of the better options.

Among your best sugars are coconut sugar, muscovado sugar, and stevia. Coconut sugar is evaporated coconut sap, with the texture of brown sugar. It is rich in phosphorus, potassium, and other natural minerals, and it has roughly half the glycemic value of cane sugar. Muscovado sugar is unrefined and comes straight from sugar cane. It looks a lot like brown sugar, but it's even more nutritious because it has been through less of a refining process. Sometimes it's called moist sugar because, well, it tends to be moist. That makes it more difficult to use in some baking, but it retains so much magnesium, potassium, calcium, and iron that it is a far better alternative. Last but not least in this category is stevia. Stevia comes from the plant **stevia rebaudiana** and belongs to the genus chrysanthemum, native to Latin America and related to our daisy. In native cultures, it is used as a sweetener in tea and to offset bitterness. I recommend it for a number

---

Off the Grid with Diabetes

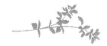

of reasons. Stevia contains glycosides—organic compounds that have a sweet taste but contain literally no calories. In fact, the extract that you are most likely to find in commercial products is 200 to 300 times more intense than refined sugar.

You can use stevia in almost any of your cooking or baking, but just remember that being sweeter than sugar, it can't be used as a one to one replacement in recipes. You may need to experiment, but remember it is powerful! Being free of all calories and carbohydrates, it gets the best glycemic rating (a zero!), so it will not cause your blood sugar to spike. In addition to being great for diabetics, it's also safe for people who are worried about yeast infections and fungal growth in their organs.

Unfortunately, stevia is not sold in the U.S. as a food additive, only as a dietary supplement. Don't worry though; it has a long proven and safe record of use in the rest of the world. It's been tested in numerous scientific studies and is not only safe but also nutritious. It has a stabilizing effect on blood glucose and has been shown to lower blood pressure and alleviate heartburn. Isn't it amazing that nature gives us something so great? The best news is that you can buy stevia plants in places that sell edible herbs, so you can truly develop your own homegrown off-the-grid supply of a healthy sugar alternative!

A little further down the list, but still acceptable, are maple syrup, brown rice syrup, and honey. Of course, maple syrup comes from the sap of the maple tree and tends to be expensive. The reason is that it takes about ten gallons of sap to produce just one quart of maple syrup (which might make you think twice about developing your own maple source). Because of the interest in maple syrup, there are a lot of artificial products, so make sure you buy 100 percent pure maple syrup!

Also acceptable is brown rice syrup, which is a rice-based sweetener. Processers add enzymes to brown rice and cook it, then filter and evaporate to create compounds that usually are

---

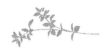

found in energy bars and health food products. This is also a good product if you are trying to go gluten-free.

Honey is of course what bees make, and it is primarily composed of fructose and glucose. Just a tablespoon of honey earns a 55 on the glycemic index, but I still consider it to be one of the better sweeteners because it contains so many healthy enzymes and minerals that support immune function. Studies in Israel proposed that honey would reduce anemia in people who are undergoing chemotherapy. At the same time, it reduced the incidence of neutropenia (low white blood counts), and we already know that honey can be applied externally to wounds and can help prevent the spread of staph infection. Not only is it healthier than refined white sugar, it has a whole host of other off-grid uses.

The last group of natural sweeteners I can recommend include turbinado sugar, fruit juice concentrate, evaporated cane juice, and agave syrup. These are not as beneficial as those I've already mentioned, but they are definitely better alternatives than the refined, processed, white sugar.

Turbinado is raw sugar, created when sugar cane is slowly boiled. It has a golden crystal-like composition and is sometimes called demarara. You're probably familiar with fruit juice concentrate, which is made from fruit juice that has had its water content reduced. Evaporated cane juice is a sweet liquid extracted from sugar cane before all the refining and bleaching occurs in the process designed to produce refined white sugar; therefore, it still contains many of its nutrients.

My personal favorite of this group is the agave syrup. It looks a lot like honey, but it comes from a plant that looks like aloe vera. However, the agave plant is native to Mexico and other parts of Central America and is the plant that mezcal (a cousin of tequila) is created from. You've probably heard of agave in this context. Anyway, agave is very sweet and thus has drawn some criticism because of its high fructose and glucose content. However,

Off the Grid with Diabetes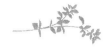

agave syrup does not normally cause a sudden rise in your blood sugar, it's far less processed than white refined sugar, and it contains natural minerals and nutrients that are lost in the alternative. So, perhaps the wise course is to use it as an alternative, but sparingly.

Sugars that I absolutely cannot recommend (in fact, that I must discourage you from using) include xylitol, high fructose corn syrup, and brown sugar. Xylitol is a synthetic sugar that is heavily processed. Some people think it is the same thing as xylem, a component to corn, but it is more closely related to sorbitol and is known to cause diarrhea.

High fructose corn syrup (HFCS) is the combination of fructose and glucose. HFCS is found in lots of our foods today such as candy bars, soda, spaghetti sauce, salad dressing, ketchup, and baked goods. The reason it is so widely used is that it is very inexpensive to produce and is extremely sweet.

With the increased use of HFCS in our processed foods, Americans are now consuming on average twelve teaspoons of HFCS on a daily basis. Scientists specializing in obesity have discovered a link between nonalcoholic fatty liver disease and the consumption of HFCS. (Liver disease is usually associated with alcoholism, so these findings were quite significant). The bottom line is that those individuals who got 20 percent or more of their daily caloric intake from HFCS began showing signs of liver disease and cellular disruption.

Scientists at the University of Pennsylvania found similarly disturbing results in a 2004 study: they discovered that eating fructose in any form, but especially HFCS, causes your body to make less leptin (the hormone that tells your brain to stop being hungry) and less insulin, thereby making it impossible for you to feel full and leading to both overeating and a reduced ability to manage the higher level of sugar in the blood.

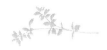# Off the Grid with Diabetes

I could continue to cite scientific studies showing the dangers of HFCS, but since you're making the decision to take your health into your hands, do your best to eliminate HFCS from your diet, wherever it is found.

Of course it is difficult to eliminate sugar from your diet completely (and who would want to?), and you might be inclined to substitute artificial sweeteners. This can be very dangerous, because most artificial sweeteners are packed with manmade chemicals, so toxic they have to get FDA approval to be sold. They have been tied to both cancer and neurological disorders. These chemicals in your body can only add to the amount of free radical damage, something already prevalent among diabetics and those with high blood sugar disorders.

What happens when these chemicals flood your body? They stimulate the cells and can actually stimulate them to death. I'm not kidding! They are called excitotoxins —exciting toxins— because as your cells get excited, they swell and can actually die. When this happens in your brain, you can get a migraine. No doubt you're familiar with acesulfame, saccharin, aspartame, sucralose, tagatose, and even the new Truvia®.

All of these sweeteners are at least partially man-made and are seen by your body as foreign invaders. Your cells don't know how to deal with foreign chemicals, which cause them to get excited. That's not a good thing. The results can be behavioral disorders, epilepsy, and cancer, among others. I know that you may want to replace sugar with something less harmful, but by and large the artificial sweetener route isn't the way to accomplish this.

Let me give you an example. Aspartame was discovered in 1965, but during testing with lab rats it was found to cause cancer. The FDA would not allow it to be used in human foods. Despite this, in 1983 the FDA approved the use of aspartame as a food additive. This, even after knowing that at high temperatures, aspartame releases a chemical that is essentially methanol, that ultimately

Off the Grid with Diabetes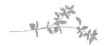

disintegrates into formaldehyde which is used to preserve dead bodies! Is it really worth the risk of having these toxic chemicals floating around in your body just for a little sweetener?

If all that's not bad enough, aspartame has been linked to lower levels of serotonin, one of the hormones that help you feel better. When lower levels of serotonin persist, you may start to experience depression, panic attacks, anxiety, hostility, agitation, insomnia, and even bipolar disorders. Why not just avoid artificial sweeteners whenever possible?

Now I want to turn your attention to the famous glycemic index (GI). The GI is based on the theory that complex carbohydrates digest more slowly in your system than simple carbohydrates, resulting in a smaller blood sugar increase. By assigning a number to each food, we can more easily predict the increase in blood sugar from consuming that food. A lot of diabetics now live by this system.

I don't think there's much danger from this diet, but I don't think that it's the silver bullet. For one, you have to constantly look things up by checking numbers and charting. Plus, since the GI of any food is based on just a single item, anything we eat that contains multiple items gets distorted. Much has been made of the pizza analogy: according to the GI diet, pizza is better for you than wheat bread because the GI for pizza is lower (because it contains cheese, which digests more slowly). I love pizza as much as anyone, but eating too much pizza will lead to obesity, high blood pressure, and certainly high blood sugar. We already know that white bread—wherever it is found—is not very good for you, and pizza made from white bread is not actually better for you than just plain whole wheat bread, even if the GI diet says it is.

A lot of critics of the GI diet point out that replicating the measurements of the diet have proven very difficult. Some people eat high GI foods and their blood sugar spikes, while

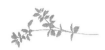

others are unaffected. Some get higher spikes from lower foods. The GI diet doesn't tell you how much insulin your body should produce, it only estimates how high your blood sugar will be two hours after you eat—but what about the effect after four or eight hours?

One of my biggest concerns with the GI diet is that testing and measurements of the GI diet were based on what happens in healthy people. Since it is diabetics that tend to need the GI diet, wouldn't it make more sense to test the GI diet with people who already have metabolic disorders and see how it affects them? Since their digestive systems are already functioning poorly and they may have a deficiency of enzymes, vitamins and minerals, it is reasonable to conclude that their bodies would respond differently.

All of these things we've covered, especially artificial sweeteners and the glycemic index, are nothing more than band-aids on the bigger problem. The problem is the food we are eating and the quantities of it. Just as the medical approach to this disease treats the symptoms rather than focusing on a reversal of the cause, so too do the diet plans, which depend on management of the blood sugar rather than dietary changes to undo the damage, restore the organs to proper function, and prevent a recurrence. That's what we're going to talk about now.

I want to share with you a way to eat well, eat healthily, and eat in a sustainable way so you can eat off grid without worrying about consulting a chart when you're in a survival situation. In a sense, foods can act like drugs in our body in that they have a cause and effect and can alter body function. So, what we consume can have a huge impact on our bodies. That's why we have the old saying "you are what you eat."

Some people are inclined to make radical dietary changes, and I want to counsel against that. I believe as humans we tend to respond better to gradual changes. If we introduce new things

Off the Grid with Diabetes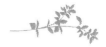

gradually, we become accustomed to them and don't even realize the difference. So here are a few big picture ideas before I get into actual food components.

Let's approach one meal at a time rather than your entire diet. If at breakfast you're accustomed to having a sugary boxed cereal from the store, let's eliminate that. Try eating some almonds, walnuts, fresh coconut, blueberries, grapefruit, or a healthy shake. Maybe choose a healthy, fiber-rich cereal that otherwise might be bland, but add one of the foods I just mentioned to it instead of sugar. I know that at first it won't taste as good, but if you try it for a few weeks, I promise you'll adjust! You won't even realize that it isn't as sugary as that cereal you used to have!

Let me share a personal example. I grew up in the South where we drink a lot of sweet tea. My mom would often add a cup of sugar to a big jar of iced tea. I loved it and drank it into adulthood. When my wife and I had kids, they started helping to make tea and would naturally, as children are want to do, add a little more sugar into the tea. Before long, there was as much as a cup and a half of refined sugar in every jug of tea! When I first started adjusting my diet, I made the switch from sweet tea to unsweetened. It was really tough. For a while there I started dropping sugar cubes into my tea. But slowly, I began weaning myself off of it. Within a month, I drank the unsweetened tea and didn't even think about it! I didn't even miss the sweetened version. In fact, one time I poured the wrong tea, drank it, and spit it out! The tea was so sweet I couldn't handle it! This was the very same tea I had been drinking for years.

I want to encourage you in the same direction with coffee (if you're a coffee drinker like me). I used to add sugar and milk to my coffee daily. When I tried to make a change, I found that black coffee was just too much. So, I kept the milk and switched to sweetener. Later, when I found out just how bad sweetener was, I dropped it. Slowly I got used to the coffee with just milk. As I learned that cow's milk wasn't good for me, I started

---

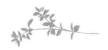

decreasing how much milk I put in the coffee. Before long, I was drinking black coffee. I still enjoyed it just as much, and I never thought about going back. But if I had tried to go all in, I never would have made it. That's just the way our bodies work.

I want to encourage you along these lines generally. Start making small adjustments to different parts of your diet. Begin with breakfast, transition to lunch, then dinner, then your snacks. If you're a late-night snacker like me, don't cut them out entirely— you'll likely fail. Try substituting healthy things you like for things that are really bad for you. If you're a soda drinker, try moving from the regular soda to the diet, and then reducing your diet intake, and then moving from diet soda to tea or coffee. Tea and coffee are both natural and good for you, after all.

Another technique I want to share with you that has been immensely valuable to me is fasting. I know what you're thinking— fasting is for old ascetic holy people. Maybe that's true. But if you are a Christian, you know that Christ commanded us to follow his example of prayer and fasting. Well, aside from the spiritual benefits, I found that fasting does wonders. Let me explain. Sometimes we eat just because we are in the habit of eating. If you normally eat at noon, you go through the motions of eating, even if you had a big breakfast or ate late and you're not even really hungry! Sometimes we eat a huge dinner even if we've snacked in the afternoon and don't really need the food. That's because our brains and bodies have been conditioned to the activity. We want to change the conditioning to our benefit.

When your life revolves around food, you've become a slave to food. I know you may not think of it all the time or obsess about it, but if you're not regularly skipping meals, then a question must be asked: does the food control you or do you control you? If you're already overweight (and most of Americans are), then it's certainly not going to hurt you to skip a few meals. But, that's not really the point. I don't want you to reverse diabetes or forestall it by starving yourself, but by disciplining yourself.

Off the Grid with Diabetes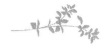

What I want to recommend is selective fasting as a means of developing stronger personal discipline and will power. When you can learn to say no to yourself and maintain that posture, you are improving your decision-making ability even in the face of discomfort (or hunger). Your body, thinking it deserves to eat, tells you that you're hungry. But in reality, it's just conditioned to eat; it doesn't really need to eat. After all, if you're five pounds overweight—and that would be a huge majority of us—you could live off that fat for days without missing a beat. That is not what I'm suggesting, however.

I fell into fasting by accident. One day I worked on a project right through lunch. It was late afternoon when I realized I was tired and had a headache. Then I remembered I hadn't eaten. The headache and the fatigue was my body complaining to me that I hadn't given it the food it was accustomed to having at the usual time. And yet, I was functioning just fine. In fact, after having a cup of coffee, I actually felt good!

I studied this issue and found that medical professionals now agree that periodic fasting is actually good for your body. It's kind of like having the system flushed every now and then. When your body is constantly busy taking in new food and digesting it, it sets aside all the maintenance tasks and extras in all the "junk drawers" of your body, thinking it will get to them later. But, on our three-or-four-meal-a -day life, the body never gets to those things. We keep it so busy all the time ingesting and digesting new foods.

So, when we fast, we trigger the body's natural mechanism to go burn off the fat that has been stored, to clean and flush things out. The body works a little harder to do this and may complain to you through a headache or fatigue, but it's not really hurting; it's just whining. Nutritionists and physicians agree that a twenty-four-hour fast can do wonders for you. I want to urge you though, that you should never abstain from drinking

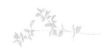

fluids, and if you are anticipating lots of vigorous physical exercise, that's not a good time to fast.

My objective here is mental and psychological training. When you consciously avoid eating and say no to yourself, you are training yourself to resist the impulse of your body. You are placing yourself in charge of your body instead of the other way around. A person who has never resisted their impulse to eat will have a very hard time with this, but a person who regularly says no to themselves will have little difficulty. It's the same as any other discipline. If you get up every morning at 6 a.m., you're accustomed to saying no to that desire to sleep in,; on the other hand, your teenager, who hates getting up and is accustomed to sleeping in until whenever you force him out of bed will probably find dealing with that impulse far more difficult.

The same is the case with food. If you have always given in to that hunger impulse, which wants to be satisfied with food, then you're not winning the argument. By selectively fasting, maybe for one meal at a time, you can start to build up a personal discipline to take charge of your body. Over time, you'll be able to skip two meals, then three. You will feel better physically, and the emotional payoff will be great as well. But the real objective is that you will have established your primacy over your impulse, so when it comes to eating a smaller portion, skipping that candy bar, or eating a double portion of vegetables, you will find it far easier than someone with no experience saying no to themselves.

Hippocrates was known to say that you should medicate yourself through your food, and that's exactly what I want to talk about now. An author I once read talked about rearranging the letters in the word "DIET" so that they spelled the word "EDIT" instead. Let's edit what we eat rather than focusing on that negative word dieting.

Off the Grid with Diabetes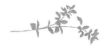

As you start to build the foundation for a nutritious food plan, you know you need to eliminate white refined sugar and artificial sweeteners. Instead, use natural sweeteners, particularly dark agave, molasses, stevia, and unrefined coconut sugar.

Where you used white flour, either all-purpose or self-rising, replace it with rice, almond, walnut, or coconut flour. Another great option, especially if you are in need of a transition from bleached white flour, would be unbleached 100 percent whole-grain flour.

Where you would normally use iodized table salt, substitute unbleached Celtic sea salt or French grey sea salt. They have all the same great flavor and are a rich source of minerals. Your pancreas and thyroid glands will appreciate the chromium, iodine, magnesium, zinc, vanadium, and iron.

If you are a snacker like me, you've got a real challenge. Commercial food processors are great at making these snack foods handy and ready to eat. If you like crackers, potato chips, or other carbohydrates that are high in salt and oil, try to substitute healthier things that are still tasty like avocados and walnuts, natural treats that contain good fats.

If you're in the habit of eating a lot of canned foods (and there's nothing wrong with canned foods, particularly in a survival situation), replace them with fresh or frozen varieties whenever possible, because canned foods bought commercially have been highly processed and have gone on a long journey with lots of wild temperature variations. Or even better, learn to can at home! It's a valuable skill to have, it's family friendly, and the result is far better than a mass-produced canned product from the grocery.

Switch your cooking from prepared foods out of a box or a plastic container to fresh, organic foods. I know that sounds like a lot of work, but we're talking about your very life here! Your local

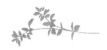

co-op, farmer's market, and even most grocery stores these days offer a wide variety of fresh foods for the growing population that is fed up with all the negative consequences of processed, commercial foods.

I know that buying fresh and organic is more expensive. Those costs can add up, but compare them to the costs of doctor's visits, medication, lost wages, or, God forbid, an early death! Just because a certain lifestyle is cheaper doesn't make it better! Plus a lot of those processed foods, especially snacks, are more expensive than you realize. As your body adjusts to the new, healthy, nutritious food, you won't find yourself as hungry throughout the day. As a result, you'll eat less. So I would suggest that the perceived increase in your food costs is actually offset by your reduced consumption.

I've already talked about how bad soda is for you, so try to eliminate soda from your diet entirely. But, if you still crave that soda feeling, try a natural soda. You can make your own soda with rich fruits that are good for you combined with some seltzer for a fresh, healthy option.

Anything with lots of transfat oils, such as margarine, lard, shortening, bacon fat, or anything with hydrogenated oil is bad for you and contributes to metabolic disorders. Instead, use grape seed oil, almond oil, extra virgin cold pressed olive oil, and coconut oil.

A replacement for candy bars, cookies, and the like would be healthy energy bars. Instead of pies and cakes, make desserts built around fruit, like raspberries, blueberries, pineapple, pomegranate, oranges, kiwi, coconut, papaya, mango, and so forth. Try to back off the sugar content or use a healthy alternative.

Anytime you have factory-farmed commercial meat and poultry products, the odds are they are infested with parasites, bacteria, antibiotics, hormones, and a myriad of dangerous chemicals. You

Off the Grid with Diabetes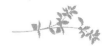

don't have to be an animal lover to be shocked by those tapes that activists sneak out of these facilities...but even worse are the conditions those animals live in and the condition of the meat preparation areas. Instead, try to eat grass-fed, free range, hormone-free products from animals that have lived a life closer to nature. This isn't a wild green strategy, but one that will almost certainly improve your health. After all, God created animals to graze in nature, not to live and die in those horrible slaughterhouses.

Now, I want to talk about your water. If you're drinking your tap water, you may be ingesting a lot more chlorine and arsenic than you imagined. Even low levels of arsenic can be bad for you. In fact, **The Journal of the American Medical Association** published a study in 2008 where they found that people with Type 2 diabetes had 26 percent higher levels of arsenic in their urine than those who are healthy. That can't be good. So, drink clean, filtered water. It's easy to buy a filter to attach to your sink or to have one professionally installed. If you're going to be developing a rainwater collection system, fabulous! Make sure the filtering and treatment methods you use are light on artificial, chemical treatments (which may only last so long anyway) and heavy on organic treatments. Some of the best long-term methods for filtering water use sand, rocks, gravel, ash, and carbon filters. As usual, nature provides the solutions for us.

If you're preparing your foods using hydrogenated fat or partially hydrogenated oils, I want to encourage you to reconsider. These chemicals have replaced pure butter in a lot of baked and fried foods. Trans fats are the result of taking pure liquid oil and treating it with chemicals in a lab to alter its state so it is more easily preserved. Trans fats are designed to be lubricants for processing food; they're not food in themselves. Basically we're talking about preservatives that help the food companies make more money, and we know that's a good thing for them, but what about for us? In the U.S. over the last few years, federal laws have begun requiring manufacturers to list the amount of

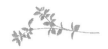 # Off the Grid with Diabetes

harmful trans fats in their products. At least now you can know when you're eating bad stuff! Be forewarned that foods filled with saturated fats and nitrates (like bacon and lard) are the very types of foods that can cause diabetes and cancer.

So, when you think about frying food, please think twice. I know that fried food tastes great, but it's terrible for you! Most people will naturally want to use cheaper oils, but these oils bear a closer resemblance to the stuff you would put in your car than the natural oils that are designed by God to aid us.

Let's review some of the different options when it comes to oil, because it won't do you much good if you try to buy the right foods but bathe them in unhealthy substances. One strategy is to alternate different oils in your cooking methods. Because oils of different origin have different levels of essential fatty acids, alternating them can give your organs a refreshing dose of nutrients. Flax oil is great oil, but if you use it exclusively, you could develop an omega-6 deficiency. Similarly, if you rely solely on sunflower oil, you could get too much omega-6. Some good and relatively inexpensive oils that come from nature are safflower, sunflower, coconut, and olive oil.

Safflower is a bright yellow flower with long spiny leaves. Oil extracted from safflower is rich in vitamin E and omega-6 acids. But, you cannot eat this oil hot because the process of warming it may kill off the benefits. I recommend it cold and in a salad dressing.

Sunflower oil is high in vitamin E and very low in bad saturated fats. You really want a brand that contains both oleic acid and linoleic acid because they are known to lower cholesterol and are also good for your heart.

Even better is coconut oil. It's solid at room temperature, which has caused some people to resist it, but it's actually great because it increases energy without having an adverse effect on your blood sugar. One of the reasons coconut oil is easier on your

Off the Grid with Diabetes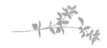

body is that the fatty acid molecules in coconut are much smaller than those in regular olive oil and even sunflower oil and are more easily digested by your body, meaning there is less leftover to be stored (as fat).

Of course, olive oil is great, and when you're going to use olive oil, you should stick with extra virgin, cold pressed olive oil, which is the cream of the crop with all the nutrients remaining. Don't fall for the temptation to buy a cheaper brand that might have a bunch of additives and substitutes. A lot of companies have begun mixing regular olive oil into very small quantities of extra virgin in an attempt to boost their profit margins. The good stuff has lots of good fatty acid, vitamins E and K, and phytosterols that help combat high cholesterol. Just because it's from Italy doesn't mean it's pure, so do some research and see which companies have a reputation for the best quality.

The next few oils I want to mention are even better for you, and as a result, they are more expensive. Begin to introduce them into your meals, perhaps not replacing the extra virgin olive oil, but balancing them at least. For example, grape seed oil is one of the best oils you can find. It's loaded with powerful antioxidants and heart-healthy compounds and may even raise your good HDL count. Flaxseed oil is also outstanding. Flax is largely cultivated for its fiber and provides essential fatty acids, which can help reduce inflammation, and it too is loaded with vitamins, minerals and nutrient alpha linoleic acids. It has a pleasant, light, nutty flavor.

Avocado oil comes from the fleshy green part of the avocado and is a fruit-based monounsaturated oil. It's rich in vitamins A, E, B1, B2 and D, low in cholesterol, and high in essential fatty acids. It's often used in high-end massage oils and has even been used to treat psoriasis and eczema. It's great for your liver and pancreas because it contains lots of glutathione, one of your body's natural astringents. By cleansing your liver of free radicals, you're helping to improve digestion. You can use avocado oil to

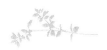

sear, sauté, even fry (please use it in limited quantities though for frying). Also, avocado oil doesn't seem to lose its nutritional value at higher temperatures.

Almond oil is another great option, especially as an alternative to butter. It's great to use in salads, desserts, and sauces. Make sure you know the difference between almond oil and extract; the extract is a concentrated flavoring you can find in any grocery store. The oil of almond, incredibly rich in nutrients, is more likely to be found in a health food store.

Hemp seed oil provides a lot of omega-3 fatty acids and contains linoleic acid. It's been around for a long time and has a wide use in cooking. It contains lots of chlorophyll and is a strong detoxifier. It might take some getting used to the color—it's a bright green! But it is low in saturated fats and is great for salads or as a finishing oil. Keep it away from high temperatures though.

Now for some oils that you should avoid at all costs: margarine and fake butter are terrible for you. They are really just chemical compounds designed for lubrication with artificial additives to make them resemble something natural. Along these same lines are cottonseed oil, processed palm oil, and hydrogenated and partially hydrogenated fats and oils. Imagine drinking automobile oil and you'll get a sense of what these oils are really made of.

Let's shift gears and talk about some foods that are the foundation of your healthy, off-grid diet. Broiled meat is great, because in the broiling process the fat tends to drip off, reducing the caloric intake. Great examples of good broiled meat options are organic beef, lamb, bison, veal, and venison. Because meat is more slowly digested, it is less of a challenge to your digestive system and therefore great for diabetics. Chicken, turkey, duck, and wild fowl are also great. Again, stick with organic and farm-raised, free-range poultry.

Fish is also high on the list, especially if it is broiled or poached. Of course you can prepare it with some extra virgin olive oil or natu-

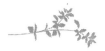

ral butter. Fresh or salt-water fish are fine, and crab is a great source of zinc. Farm-raised commercial fish should be avoided as they are usually fed a chemical diet, including a lot of antibiotics that you don't need in your system.

Eggs are also fine in any style, but I strongly encourage you to stick with free-range and organic eggs. Try not to fry them in hot oil; poaching is a great alternative.

We've talked about milk products before, so I'll only touch on it here. If you are going to use cow's milk, try to stick with organic, locally raised cattle. Try to find sheep's milk or goat products. Organic whole milk, cream, butter, cheese, and even quark, kefir and yogurt are acceptable.

On your new plan, vegetables will be the primary source of your carbohydrates, so you need to begin working into your meals the following, all of which are safe:

- Arugula
- Asparagus
- Beet greens
- Broccoli
- Brussels sprouts
- Cabbage
- Cauliflower
- Celery
- Chinese cabbage
- Cilantro
- Collards
- Cucumbers
- Dandelion greens
- Eggplant
- Endive
- Garlic
- Green beans
- Green onions
- Kale

- Kohlrabi
- Leeks
- Lettuce
- Mushrooms
- Muskmelon
- Mustard greens
- Onions (raw)
- Parsley
- Pumpkin
- Radish sprouts
- Radishes
- Sauerkraut
- Spinach
- Squash
- Tomatoes
- Turnip greens
- Turnips
- Watercress
- Wax beans

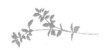

In limited quantities—don't make these a daily affair—you can consume cantaloupe, honeydew melon, watermelon, and strawberries. Also permitted in limited amounts are soybeans, cooked onions, rutabagas, and green and black olives. I also like lemons, limes, avocados, pickles, and capers.

Except where I've specifically identified fruit, it should be avoided because of the high sugar content, at least until you're off medicine and your body has recovered (and for most people that will happen). If you're worried about sources of vitamin C and don't have a supplement, then I would choose grapefruit, wild blueberries, strawberries, papaya, and hard kiwi.

A lot of sources will recommend nuts, but they can contain relatively high amounts of carbohydrates in a concentrated form, which can be fattening. Cheese would be a better option, as it is much lower in carbohydrates. However, cold-pressed nut oils are okay because they are a concentrated source of key nutrients that can actually help reverse the disease. One of my favorites would be cold-pressed pumpkin seed oil, which helps speed fat burning in your cells.

One of the areas we can get creative in keeping your food tasty while actually turning back the clock on diabetes is with select condiments. Pickles (as long as they are unsweetened), mustard, organic vinegar, and horseradish are all great. In fact, high-quality vinegar not only stimulates digestion but aids in mineral absorption, something many diabetics really need.

I want to highlight some foods that are particularly good for diabetics. Whether vegetable or tubular, artichokes are superb because they gently aid kidney function, help to flush poisons from the liver, and contain a compound that aids in liver cell regeneration. In Europe, artichokes are used for jaundice, and since all diabetics have compromised livers, artichokes should be on the menu. Artichokes are also naturally very dense in vitamins and minerals and provide a great source of magnesium and

Off the Grid with Diabetes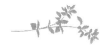

folic acid. They also contain iodine, copper, zinc, magnesium, calcium, phosphorus, iron, potassium, and manganese.

But the best part of the artichoke is the inulin. As much as 30 percent of each artichoke is inulin, which is of immense value to diabetics because it is a carbohydrate that puts no stress on your pancreas; it does not cause the release of insulin. It's kind of natural insulin itself, unlike most carbohydrates that agitate pancreatic function. Artichokes also contain cynarin, which boosts liver function and protects it against toxins. Cynarin is believed to stimulate the production of bile, which helps to explain why artichokes are credited with lowering cholesterol and triglyceride levels.

When we discussed alternatives to unhealthy oils, we mentioned oil from avocado. The avocado is another one of those superfoods that diabetics can enjoy because it is rich in nutrients, essential fatty acids, and monounsaturates. It is often attacked because of the fat content, but natural fats are a good thing. In studies in Australia, cardiologists have demonstrated that the regular intake of avocados actually improves heart function and lowers cholesterol. Avocados offer nutrients and minerals in exceptionally concentrated values. You'll find biotin, thiamine, niacin, beta-carotene, folic acid, pyridoxine, and vitamin E in avocados.

Another diabetic superfood is cod liver and cod liver oil. This food delivers pure, natural vitamin A. Since diabetics often suffer from the inability to properly metabolize vitamin A (beta carotene), consuming it in a ready-to-use form (as it is found in cod liver) is critical. Vitamin A helps to protect tissues from the effects both of toxic damage and age. It also helps organs develop strong epithelial cell lining.

Since diabetics usually suffer from digestive problems, food that is naturally easily digestible helps diabetics overcome their deficiency. That's why I strongly recommend fatty fishes. Another

---

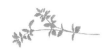

advantage is that fatty fishes rarely provoke allergic reactions, which is perhaps due to the prevalence of omega-3 fatty acids, which are more easily digested than animal fats. Omega-3 fats help to reduce inflammation and tend to thin the blood, which is why they are recommended for fighting heart disease, strokes, and high blood pressure. Because of these natural properties, they facilitate good cellular operation and growth. Because human cells are built around membrane and fluid operations, fish fats help them to remain more lubricated and pliant, and therefore more flexible and resistant to damage. Since aging, dysfunctional cells are often stiff ones, it's easy to see why keeping cells flexible and well-lubricated can have a beneficial effect, not just on your general health, but in organs that are otherwise stressed by metabolic disorders.

Another food that is virtually predigested is yogurt. As you already know, yogurt is very different from milk, being curdled and clumpy, the result of protein and fats already having been processed. Of course, I recommend goat or sheep's yogurt over bovine products. You'll find they are far richer than cow's products and are much less likely to provoke an allergic response Because yogurt is more easily digested, the nutrients within can be absorbed at a rate of three times other animal products. Milk and cheese normally require a great deal of human enzymes to digest, placing a strain on the digestive system, but yogurt skips this process because the enzyme process has already been performed by the microbes that result in that clumpy condition. Further, the fat content makes the yogurt gentler and also slows down digestion, smoothing out the spike in blood sugar you might otherwise expect. Additionally, the sugar content in yogurt is already fermented, reducing the stress and strain on the digestive system that is otherwise involved in converting that sugar (which we call lactose). That's why if you are going to consume milk, it is actually better to avoid low fat or skim milk, because you have removed the very barrier that aids digestion (the fat) and exposed the organs and arteries to the harsh sugar.

Off the Grid with Diabetes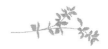

Rice bran and rice polish are great food concentrates and are among the most nutritionally dense foods a diabetic can consume. When you eat rice bran, you are getting bran and polish, but you are also consuming starch that is otherwise not desirable. However, the density of nutrients in these two concentrates is almost unmatched. They contain an enormous amount of B vitamins, fiber, minerals, phytochemicals, amino acids, fatty acids, and cofactors, all of which are natural. Your body utilizes all these compounds efficiently and easily. Rice bran is a great food just for the B vitamin content.

Another excellent superfood is the radish because it is rich in phytochemicals and sulfur compounds that stimulate digestion and boost organ efficacy. The heat of the radish stimulates digestive juices, which diabetics are often low on. Of course, because the heat is the source of the healing power, the hotter the radish, the better. Radishes also contain a lot of trace minerals that they draw from the soil they're grown in, including selenium, a powerful, immunity-boosting mineral known to combat cancer.

Like radishes, onions are great medicinal food and one of the most diverse food sources for diabetics. Onions actually contain a hormone that mimics the effect of insulin in the body and oils that have a germicidal-like effect in the circulatory system. Onions also contain vitamin C and sulfur (which is great for healthy skin, hair, and nails) and, like radishes, tend to stimulate healthy digestive action. This is particularly the case with heavy animal meats that otherwise challenge digestion. Onions also have an antiseptic function that mitigates against infection.

Since high heat can destroy many of these properties, onions offer the best value when they are served raw. In fact, cooking can caramelize the natural sugar in onions leading to a spike in blood sugar! Because onions are high in carbohydrates, you should moderate your intake until your blood sugar is stabilized naturally. Again, the carbohydrate value increases with cooking.

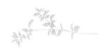

Green onions have the lowest carb value, with Vidalia, Spanish, and red onions at the high end of the scale.

Garlic is one of my favorite anti-diabetic foods, not just because it adds such a great flavor to so many foods, but also because it lowers blood sugar and blood fat levels. It can even cause blood sugar levels to fall too rapidly, so be careful! Garlic is also great for your cardiovascular health because it lowers triglycerides and cholesterol. Garlic can help prevent fat from being deposited in your arteries, thereby reducing your risk of heart and arterial disease. As with the other vegetables, garlic is best served fresh, because cooking and processing can strip so many healthy things from it and add unknown quantities of harsh additives.

One of the best green options you have is parsley. It has more vitamins, proteins, and minerals than just about any other vegetable, and the great thing is that it can be grown just about anywhere in the world! Parsley was even used in ancient times: Roman physicians used it as a natural diuretic and to treat urinary disorders. In Britain it has been used to dissolve kidney stones, and some herbalists believed it helps to reverse arthritis. Parsley is rich in protein, containing as much protein as the equivalent amount of corn meal. It contains three times as much vitamin C (by weight) as does an orange. It has more folic acid than broccoli and has three times more magnesium per ounce than whole grain. Of course, as a dark green vegetable, it is also a great source of carotenes and flavonoids.

Another ancient food that doubles as a curative agent is the dandelion green. It has been used to treat liver disorders for more than a millennium. The juice extract of dandelion is a particularly powerful agent and is a top source of natural calcium, potassium, sodium, phosphorus, and magnesium and helps to neutralize stomach acidity. Some of the sugars in the dandelion are now understood to be inulin, the compound that simulates the natural process of insulin. In addition to helping aid liver function, dandelion has a curative action against eczema, blood

Off the Grid with Diabetes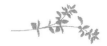

disease, anorexia, congestive heart failure, and even arthritis. Think twice the next time you want to use harsh pesticides to exterminate dandelions from your lawn!

Another spicy and beneficial food that should be a regular part of any diabetic diet is the watercress. One of the hottest of all vegetables, the watercress helps to improve the function of liver cells by stimulating the flow of bile. Bile works in the liver by flushing out toxins that tend to gather there as well as assisting in the breakdown of fats and proteins. The source of watercress' heat is the natural sulfur, which works like an intestinal tonic as well as forming part of the chemical chain in the synthesis of numerous hormones, among which are insulin. Many researchers also believe these same heat-producing compounds are cancer preventatives as well.

Another spice-producing plant with some heat that is an excellent tonic for the diabetic's stressed system is coriander, also known by its Spanish name of cilantro. Cilantro contains a number of natural chemicals that stimulate liver and digestive function as well as boosting the metabolic rate, aiding in the burning of fat. If you're burning fat, there is less fat to be stored, so in a roundabout way you're helping to prevent diabetes, while at the same time helping those processes that are usually affected by diabetic organ failure. Cilantro leaves are widely available, and of course this is an herb you can also grow yourself—ideal for an off-grid spice. The leaves are also an excellent source of potassium, better even than oranges or bananas. There are a great many tasty dishes that cilantro works well in too, from traditional Mexican fare to Mediterranean dishes.

At the other end of the spectrum is one of the most famous natural diabetic treatments, the blueberry! Blueberries contain lots of natural pancreatic and liver boosters, but it is only the wild blueberries that can be counted on to perform this function. In particular is the bilberry species of blueberry, which has been documented to help with a wide range of disorders,

---

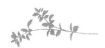

including Reynaud's Syndrome, poor circulation, hemorrhoids, nose health, diabetic retinopathy, varicose veins, fragile blood vessels, and high blood pressure.

If you're suffering from some diabetic-related eye damage, you may be thrilled to learn that bilberries have been shown to help with photosensitivity, glaucoma, retinal disorders, nearsightedness, and poor night vision. The seeming miracle food is so effective because of the wide range of flavonoids and enthocyanins. Researchers have found that the leaves are particularly high in these compounds, so consider making tea from these leaves for a real boost to your system.

I've already mentioned how cheese can be an ideal food for diabetics because it contains very little or no carbohydrates while having a lot of protein. However, because of the problems with cow's milk, I recommend feta cheese, produced from the milk of goats or sheep. Feta cheese is easy to digest and is a low stress food, therefore failing to cause problems with the digestive system. Just make sure before you embark on a shopping spree that the feta cheese is organic and truly made from goat or sheep's milk.

Traditional diabetic diets urge avoidance of anything with sugar content. You'll notice that my recommendation is a little different, including fruits that may be high in sugar and other items that might not otherwise be on the list. I believe the trade off is a good one, that the good things in these fruits and carbs are necessary for a balanced diet, but I am also assuming that you will follow my recommendation and include lots of herbs and spices in your meals, which will more than counteract the natural sugars you consume, while also aiding in digestion and organ cleansing.

Generally speaking, foods that are always good include fresh meat and poultry, cream cheese, eggs, butter, greens, broccoli, cabbage, cauliflower, cress, cucumbers, mushrooms, asparagus, celery, radishes, vinegar, pickles, egg custard, salad oil, olives, and nuts.

Off the Grid with Diabetes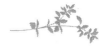

Foods that you really should avoid at all costs include white bread, biscuits, white rice, sago, tapioca, white pasta, potatoes, carrots, parsnips, beets, peas, pastry, and of course, processed sweets.

As your blood sugar starts to get under control, I can recommend adding back to your diet things like whole coarse grains, wild rice, brown rice, potato skins, kiwi, watermelon, honeydew, strawberries, blueberries, blackberries, organic peanuts and peanut butter (as long as there is no hydrogenated component), lima beans, wild honey, sour oranges, peaches, and pears.

I want to spend a few moments reviewing some of the best dietary uses of herbs and spices. Although you have undoubtedly heard of some of these, few Americans have any idea of just how versatile and powerful a few herbs are in just about any dish. The beauty of this is that many of these herbs and spices are things you may be able to grow in your own garden.

I always recommend that any source of seeds come from all-natural, non-genetically modified sources and from a dealer with a good reputation. Additionally, you should always insist on organic and non-irradiated herbs and spices. Ideal are those that are wild or mountain grown. The commercial alternative may be contaminated with pesticides, radioactive particles, and other residues, which, if not within the herb itself, may have contaminated other surfaces somewhere along the process. Many companies produce multiple lines of products, and therefore, one line can easily infect across multiple lines.

Most of the spices I am going to recommend can be consumed freely because they have insulin-boosting properties, are all-natural, and also offer germicidal properties. The benefits to your health can be immense.

One of the most famous herbs is well-known as a medicine but is also one of the finest herbal additions to food you can imagine. I'm talking about basil! It's easy to digest and is a great source of

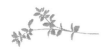

calcium and potassium. Of course, it goes great with tomato and cheese dishes and is a wonderful compliment to olive oil, soups, and pastries.

Another herb with an ancient history of medicinal use is black seed. It has been used to treat a wide range of diseases, including breathing disorders and intestinal problems, and it adds flavor to any dish, but particularly meats, casseroles, and cheese-based meals. I love it in hot breads and buns, and the oil of black seed contains plant sterols, which are known to be cancer preventives.

Caraway is great to add in soups, salad dressings, yogurt, cottage cheese, and even in hard cheese and feta cheese. I also like chives in this capacity, and of course you can mix chives into quiche, eggs, and a wide range of salads.

Capers are also great for use with salads or when mixed into cheese-based dips or avocado components. It's a great garnish for salads and vegetable dishes, and it is both a good source of potassium and helps to stimulate the flow of bile.

One of the most ancient medicinal foods is cinnamon. Hippocrates used it as a medicine, and even today in many rural cultures cinnamon is in wide use. Cinnamon greatly assists with the digestion of sugars and starches and improves the taste of poultry and rice dishes. Just experiment—you'll be surprised at all the possibilities.

Cumin is another spice with a long history of use across several cultures. It is a great digestive aid and a wonderful liver tonic. Cumin is very common in Mexican-style dishes and adds a rich flavor to any fatty dish, including those with beef, eggs, poultry, and cheese.

Dill is a great source of calcium, potassium, and magnesium, and horseradish is a wonder food when it comes to digestion, ideal for steaks, fish, and seafood. Fennel stems and bulbs are also great for stomach disorders and when raw can be used in place of celery.

Off the Grid with Diabetes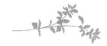

Mint has a wide range of uses and is a well-known digestive aid. Mustard, being highly acidic, boosts metabolism and can assist in weight loss. It's also a mild antibiotic. Oregano is one of the more versatile and powerful spices. Truly wild oregano is a great germicide, which has been proven in repeated lab tests.

Cloves also have a long history and are known to have significant antiseptic properties and can even be used as an anesthetic because they can reduce or numb pain. The oil of cloves is a concentrated painkiller and is commonly used for toothaches. Cloves are also a great source of antioxidant phenols and are another source of manganese.

Poppy seeds are a great source of fatty acids and can be mixed in with cheese dishes, with yogurt and pine nuts, or with hot vegetables or soups.

Another wonderful aid for digestion is rosemary because it stimulates digestion of fatty milk products. Sage also works in this capacity. Sesame seeds can be used in baking and as a great addition to stews, soups, and casseroles. It's best to add them at the end of the cooking process so the high heat doesn't destroy the nutritional value. They're a rich source of tryptophan, and the oil of sesame is a great emollient.

I've not tried to provide an exhaustive use of all these herbs because you can easily search the web for recipes that include these ingredients in significant amounts. Remember, the more you begin to adapt your menu to include these natural superfoods, the faster your body will begin to heal and grow. At the same time, if you're working on your own survival garden, you'll want to immediately incorporate as many of these herbs and spices into your master plan as possible. Congratulations and good eating!

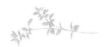 Off the Grid with Diabetes

Chapter Six:

Natural, Off-Grid Supplements for Diabetic Health

As we've discussed in previous chapters, the current pharmaceutical approach to managing high blood sugar condemns the victim to a lifetime of dependency on ever higher doses of dangerous, synthetic chemicals. While insulin may help to depress the symptoms, the disease continues to ravage the body, taking a deadly toll on the organs and contributing to the all-too-common deterioration in diabetics.

As we contemplate a life-changing event that could eliminate insulin as an option, we will uncover safer and more effective natural therapies that will heal our tissues and organs, cleanse internally, normalize digestion, and allow for the absorption of critical minerals and nutrients that are often lacking in the diabetic body. Additional benefits of the diet we outlined previously and the natural supplements you'll discover in this chapter include the cleansing of fungal and germ infestation, a restoration of hormone balance, and improvement in blood and mental performance. In other words, a far better life!

One of the most important components to your supplement therapy going forward is spice extract. They are powerful blood sugar regulators because they are natural forms of insulin that are far safer and more effective than artificial insulin. They are potent, free of dangerous side effects, and pose no risk of organ damage.

One of the reasons that spice extracts are so beneficial is their ability to kill germs, and often the diabetic is severely infected because his immune system is on life support. Among the threats commonly faced by diabetics are fungi, yeasts,

---

bacteria, parasites, and viruses. Potent spice extracts have been proven to kill both bacteria and fungi while at the same time lowering blood sugar levels. What a powerful combination! As with all my recommendations, it is critical that the source is taken into consideration: you want to insist on organically grown, non-genetically modified sources that have not been subjected to irradiation or mixed in with other commercially prepared spices. This will help to ensure you do not unintentionally ingest chemicals that harm your body.

One of my favorite spices is cumin, which has been used for thousands of years. It's a rich source of phenolic compounds, which are enormously effective in aiding digestion because they are antifungal. One of the reasons cumin is so great at combating fungal infections is because it is great at destroying mycotoxins which are known to be a leading cause of human illnesses and a primary infectant of grains, causing allergies and intolerance in humans. The reason cumin is found in nature with these great properties is that plants need protection from fungal infection and produce these substances as a result. So when we consume them, we inherit the same resistance. Additionally, cumin introduces glutathione into our system. Glutathione has become increasingly popular in recent years as scientists have been able to isolate the compound and test it on volunteers and athletes.

Cinnamon is another powerful supplement. Of course, I discussed cinnamon as an additive to your diet, but in this context I want to review its role as a medicinal supplement. Cinnamon is native to Sri Lanka and Madagascar and is derived from the dried internal bark of the cinnamon tree. It can be found in similar forms in China. The best way to obtain cinnamon is to buy fresh sticks and grind them yourself as you need them.

Extracts of cinnamon have been proven to reduce blood sugar level, and it has even been shown to neutralize the noxious effect of sugar and white flour in tests. One of the miracles of cinnamon is that its very sweetness helps to combat the effect of sugar.

Off the Grid with Diabetes

The active ingredient in cinnamon is polyphenol, which mimics insulin. Because it is naturally occurring, the body easily recognizes it, therefore negating the need for the production of more insulin. Although it's great to add cinnamon to food, anyone who is seriously diabetic needs cinnamon in greater doses, so taking a supplement which contains cinnamon along with cumin (and the fenugreek we will discuss shortly) is one way to flood your system. In our review I will discuss other methods.

Fenugreek is the final spice critical to building a spice-based medicinal treatment. Fenugreek aids in the burning of blood sugar and therefore directly and naturally lowers blood sugar, almost as rapidly as naturally produced insulin. Because it increases the number of insulin receptors on the cells, it is also building a long-term defensive mechanism for the body to manage itself, rather than just acting as a short-term stimulant, as chemicals do.

Among Type 1 diabetics, fenugreek has proven enormously powerful. In a study at Hyderabad's National Institute of Nutrition, fenugreek in the daily diet led to a 54 percent decrease in urinary glucose excretion. In other words, this spice helped to cut in half the amount of sugar that Type 1 diabetics were excreting. That's enormous! On top of that, significant reductions in cholesterol and triglyceride levels were also observed, reflecting an improvement in the condition of the blood and organ function.

One of the critical points I need you to remember is that the combination of these three ingredients has proven far more effective than any of them used alone. So, what I recommend is you find a good, reliable source of supplements that contain cumin, cinnamon, and fenugreek in abundance, and stockpile that as part of your survival kit. Additionally, do your best to purchase fresh sources, grind them fresh, and produce your own herbal treatment. If you have the capacity to explore growing these on your own, then even better! In the interim, take the

---

precautions you can to store them and most importantly, begin implementing them into your life.

Although not a spice, another critical medicinal that is also edible is kelp. Kelp is a great source of natural vitamin A, B, and C. It is also loaded with minerals your body needs, including sodium, iodine, and chlorine. Kelp is known to stimulate your fatty-acid based metabolism, which helps to burn excess fat. In addition, kelp boosts thyroid function and has even been shown to have a modest effect on the treatment of those with thyroid disorders. Crude kelp can be found in multi-vitamins, in special kelp tablets, and in some markets can even be found freshly dried and ground.

These fresh sources are best because the processing involved in creating vitamins often strips out the iodine, which doesn't survive the heating process. If you live near the coast and want to get kelp from one of the kelp farms on the continental shelf, I want to warn you that many of these sources have been shown to be infected with mercury, copper, cadmium, lead, and arsenic due to runoff from rivers laden with industrial pollution.

The best sources for natural kelp are in the far north of Canada, close to the Arctic Ocean. I know you can't go on an Arctic expedition just to find good kelp, but use your discretion now that you are in the market for kelp, looking for suppliers who are aware of these risks. Of course, the Japanese are big consumers of kelp and so that market may offer opportunities for you as well.

Because diabetes is a whole-body disease, we have to treat the mineral deficiencies that can complicate the effects of high blood sugar and organ failure. At the top of that list is chromium. In plants, chromium is used for starch and sugar metabolism. In our bodies, the presence of chromium can be tied directly to our tolerance of glucose. As with everything else, there is naturally occurring chromium, which is absorbed and metabolized by plants, and a synthetic type that is far more difficult for our

Off the Grid with Diabetes

bodies to accept. Naturally occurring chromium is easily found in whole grains.

Some spices are also high in chromium, such as turmeric, which gives curry powder that rich yellow color. Chromium is also found in black pepper, coriander, and red sour grape powder. This last source of chromium should also be a foundation of your medicinal herbal treatment. Crude red sour grape is foreign to many in the West, but it has been used in the Middle East for centuries as a treatment for everything from angina, heart failure, coronary heart disease, high cholesterol, and high blood pressure. Crude red sour grape is different than the extract from grape seed, because the sour grape is a special, mountain-grown source with no chemical additives or pesticides.

The relevance of mountain-grown sources is that drainage from pesticide-based farming and residential, commercial, and industrial runoff has not polluted the soil on a mountain like they do in valleys. On the sides of mountains, there is no runoff and no dangerous chemicals to seep into the soil. The grape is sun-dried on the vine and has the chance to develop nutrients. When the herbal treatment is being developed, it is often the entire vine, leaf, and grape that are used. Very little of this product ever makes it to market.

Other grape seed extracts are on the market, but I cannot recommend them, because the process of extraction involves the use of methyl chloride, hexane, and formaldehyde. The seeds are usually developed from commercially grown seeds, which means pesticides are involved, and while the grape can be washed, the seeds themselves have absorbed the chemicals and cannot be cleansed of them.

Red sour grape powder is free of these dangers, because it is only exposed to the sun and human grinding rather than the harsh and dangerous chemicals. As a circulatory aid, it nourishes the heart and arteries and improves their flexibility. It is a great

Off the Grid with Diabetes

source of natural chromium, and as little as three teaspoons of the powder will, on its own, supply all your daily requirements of chromium. Of course, other food sources of chromium exist, including yeast, liver, kidney, nuts, and seeds, but these don't form a very high percentage of the average American diet.

Red sour grape also contains potassium, another mineral that many diabetics are deficient in. The taste is sour as the name implies, and for some it can take some getting used to, but for others the powder can have an almost addictive component.

Another mineral that is essential for diabetics, particularly in a curative mode, is magnesium. Magnesium helps to stabilize heart function and also reduces the incidence of depression and helps to improve pain tolerance. Unfortunately, magnesium is often stripped out in the processing of many of our food products. Other foods that are naturally rich in magnesium don't play a large role in our typical diet. Examples of these include unrefined grains, nuts, and green vegetables. If you're on diuretics, blood pressure pills, steroids, estrogens, or diabetic medications, you may unknowingly be triggering a magnesium deficiency since these medications can strip the magnesium already present in your body.

Unfortunately, calcium has a natural opposition to magnesium, so if you're supplementing with calcium, you may be worsening the problem. One way to combat this is to reduce your calcium supplementation and increase your natural intake of magnesium. One sign of a magnesium deficiency is muscle cramping. However, you may also notice anxiety, restless leg syndrome, trouble sleeping, low blood pressure, an abnormal heart rhythm, and poor nail or hair growth.

Iron is another mineral that is essential to proper organ function that many of us are deficient in. Because iron is fundamental to enzyme reactions and helps to deliver oxygen to our cells, it's easy to see how in a diabetic body (where the cells are already

Off the Grid with Diabetes

struggling with glucose) to have an oxygen deficiency can easily trigger a cascade of problems. Since your intestines are often the storage system of iron, a healthy digestive system is critical. As we already know, many diabetics have a poorly functioning digestive tract, so while we're correcting that problem, we'll want to supplement with iron. You may be deficient in iron if you are cranky, depressed, or have trouble concentrating. Another sign is unusually weak fingernails or a fast heartbeat (without exertion). Before you start in on an iron supplement, do your best to find more iron-rich food sources, such as lean meat, liver, eggs, kale, spinach, turnip greens, whole grain breads, raisins, and molasses.

One final mention in the mineral category is vanadium. Although your body only needs a tiny amount of vanadium, it will also notice the slightest deficiency. If you have high cholesterol and high blood sugar, you are much more likely to have a deficiency of vanadium. Of course, if you can cure the high blood sugar through other means, the vanadium deficiency may resolve itself. Because vanadium can be a stress on the kidneys, I really would prefer you not supplement artificially and instead rely on natural food sources to get this supplement, which exists in sufficient quantities for most people. Foods that are good sources for vanadium include whole grains, seafood, seeds, mushrooms, dill, olive oil, beans, carrots, greens, garlic, lettuce, and pepper.

All these minerals are fundamental to proper organ function and are best achieved through proper diet and natural organic supplements.

The next category of supplements may be a stretch for you: I want to encourage you to begin drinking phytonutrients! A phytonutrient is derived from plant-based nutrients like beta-carotene, vitamin C, and other rich, green plants. I know, it doesn't sound great, but these health tonics are packed with essential vitamins, minerals, amino acids, enzymes, chlorophyll, micronutrients, and antioxidants.

Off the Grid with Diabetes

These green drinks are really liquid medicinal treatments, not food substitutes, which is why I'm mentioning it here and not in the food section. Some people will try to fool you into thinking that it is food, but you'll realize pretty quickly this is not something you'll ever confuse for a good meal. But, if you want to reverse the effects of diabetes, this is a quick way to restore your body's health. These medicinal drinks I'll recommend can provide exponentially greater nutritional value than your multivitamins. It's also a great way to boost your intake of fruits and vegetables.

So, I want to introduce a single-celled, blue-green algae called spirulina. Spirulina is a rich source of protein and has almost twice as much protein as you'll find in beef. Spirulina is also a great source of potassium, calcium, chromium, iron, copper, zinc, magnesium, manganese, selenium, sodium, and phosphorus. Spirulina also contains carotenoids, beta-carotenes, B vitamins, and vitamins E and K in abundance. Spirulina has also been known to ease depression. After mother's milk, this algae is one of the best sources of gamma linolenic acid you can get. You can find spirulina online and in health food stores in a variety of forms. The closer you can get to fresh organic sources of spirulina, the better.

Another green superfood that I want to recommend for blood sugar control and overall body health is chlorella. It is also a single-celled algae, and it gets its name from the high amount of chlorophyll it contains. Chlorella causes a reduction in body fat, serum total cholesterol, and blood sugar levels by boosting metabolism and improving insulin pathways. Chlorella can eliminate toxins from your digestive tract, liver, and colon, cleaning out pesticides, herbicides, alcohol, polychlorbiphenyls, and heavy metals such as cadmium, arsenic, lead, and mercury. That's a lot of housecleaning!

The final green superfood I want to mention is barley grass. Barley grass looks like regular, green grass, and it is high in vitamins B, C, and E. It also has a powerful free radical scavenger known as SOD that is believed to fight cancer, inflammatory disease, and even pancreatitis. Studies have shown that its anti-inflammatory properties are so powerful that it may work in treating rheumatoid arthritis, so if the diabetic condition has led to inflamed organs, this is the perfect treatment.

The best way to utilize these three greens is in a combination supplement that includes all three. Putting them in liquid form makes it far easier for your body to digest because compact pills formed under high pressure are alien to the body. We all know that if you drink fluid the body deals with it more quickly and efficiently than solid foods. So, I would recommend that you locate a reliable source for these three greens and put them into a drink you can consume daily as part of your rehabilitation and health regimen.

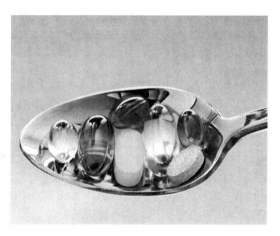

The health benefits are enormous. These green drinks can reverse Type 2 diabetes by protecting the pancreas and insulin-producing cells. They can protect your eyesight because they are abundant in carotenoids. They can provide an energy boost and overcome chronic fatigue because they are loaded in B vitamins. Green drinks will improve the growth of your nails and hair and support glucose metabolism.

Because of the natural iodine, selenium, and iron, thyroid performance is enhanced. You should experience a reduction in infection because of the antiviral activity of blue-green algae, and the folic acid and phytochemicals can even reduce the risk of cancer.

Because spirulina can block the production of interleukin 4, your hay fever symptoms may be reduced. Sneezing, runny nose, and itchy eyes could be something of the past! Plus, you are reducing the risk of cardiovascular disease, and the prevalence of the chelators in your system means neuropathic damage can be reduced. Since many of these green drinks contain probiotics, you can discourage the growth of pathogenic bacteria in your gut, helping to promote the growth of natural intestinal flora that is often destroyed by harsh medicines.

I hope you're convinced as to the health benefits of these green drinks and how they can immediately begin the process of cleansing your tissues and organs and helping restore your body to its optimum natural state. But there are a few recommendations I'd like to make at the same time.

The effect of these drinks is powerful, but sometimes it will take your body time to heal, adjust, and produce the new mitochondrial cells that benefit you. In the process, you will experience changes akin to healing, and it may not at first seem that things are better. Change is often difficult, so I want you to commit to giving this new regimen a full thirty days before changing anything else. Part of the reason for this is that because these drinks will cause your body to begin operating more efficiently, you will find that any kind of medication will have a stronger effect on you. For example, an antihypertensive medication may lead to dizziness or lightheaded bouts.

Those symptoms indicate that you should reduce your dosage and also that the green drinks are having their intended effect. I'm not suggesting you drink these drinks because they taste wonderful—I'll go ahead and admit that they don't—but because of the powerful cleaning and building effect. It would be best to start out easy; if you're using a recipe off the web, consider trying only half the concentrate to water ratio for a few weeks before going with the full dose. That will help your body adjust.

Off the Grid with Diabetes

Because these natural flavors are so foreign to our processed-food conditioned taste buds, you might find that the flavor isn't desirable. Consider mixing in some organic apple or grape juice for a few days. But do so sparingly, just enough to mask the taste, but not enough to create a great-tasting drink. This is medicine, remember? If you go this route, begin diluting it a little every day to wean yourself off. Of course, you should be using these drinks with pure, filtered water and not chemically cleaned sewage product from your city or county wastewater treatment facility.

Another thing I want to caution you about is changing all sorts of routines at once. Don't change your other medications or supplements. Do one thing at a time and see how your body reacts, and don't use a day or a week as a test period—use the full month to let things settle. So, establish your plan and begin executing things one at a time. The same goes for your diet—don't go whole hog, but start making one change at a time; this is easier on your body and also psychologically easier for you to tackle.

If you are buying the greens in any form other than fresh or dried—for example, in powder or tablet form—make sure that the ingredients are all natural and all organic. You might find some artificial sweeteners in these drinks! That defeats the whole purpose! Fortunately, you can do plenty of research online on most products and may even find the right product online at a better price than you could in a health food store that must pay for expensive retail space and employees to man the store.

Once you're a month into your new diet and new green drink supplement, the next most important change to make is the addition of vitamin D, and specifically D3. Vitamin D3 has been shown to increase insulin sensitivity by up to 60 percent in clinical tests, better even than metformin! Imagine that for the last fifteen years the pharmaceutical industry and most doctors have known that this simple vitamin is more effective than the leading diabetes drug, and I bet you've not heard about it until now! Remember, there's only so much money to be made in natural cures....

Vitamin D is fatty, so it gets into all the nooks and crannies of your body with great antioxidants that other vitamins and some chemically designed supplements cannot. Since most diabetics are deficient in vitamin D anyway, this is a must-have supplement. In fact, among children with vitamin D deficiency, there is a substantially higher risk of developing Type 1 diabetes. So don't hold back on the vitamin D supplements!

One of the best ways to get your vitamin D is naturally—in the sun. Just ten or twenty minutes a day can get you a great dose of the best kind of vitamin D your body needs, and in the preferred form. Of course, not everyone can get outside for sun, and during the winter or in regions that don't have a lot of sun, you will have to look to foods and supplements.

One of the best sources of vitamin D3 is cod liver oil, either in liquid form or soft gel form. D3 is also known as cholecalcifero, and you may find it listed this way. You can start with 4,0000 to 5,000 IU per day for the first two weeks, and then reduce your intake to 2,000 per day for another two weeks, or until your vitamin D levels are normal. How do you know when they have stabilized? Well, you can ask your doctor to test, or you can order a home testing kit. These can be purchased online for about $65, and the instructions and results are easy to understand. If you have a kidney or liver problem, you'll want to consult your doctor before you take any supplements, but particularly vitamin D, which can tax your liver and kidneys.

Some medications strip your body of vitamin D, so you'll want to review things in your household to make sure you're not taking one step forward and two backward. Acid blockers, antacids, anticonvulsants, budesonide, butalbital-based drugs, calcium channel blockers, cholestyramine, colestipol, flunisolide, fluticasone, ketoconazole, isoniazid, laxatives containing magnesium citrate, mineral oil, olestra, orlistat, raloxifene, rifampin, steroids, valproic acid, and statin cholesterol drugs all tend to deplete your natural vitamin D.

Off the Grid with Diabetes

The next step I want to encourage is to increase your fiber intake gradually. Even diabetics on a relatively poor high-carb diet begin to see improvements in their insulin resistance merely by increasing their natural fiber intake.

Fiber naturally occurs in beans, vegetables, grains, and fruits. The average American gets about fifteen grams of fiber daily, but we really need twenty-five to thirty grams. Fiber is either soluble or insoluble. We need both kinds of fiber, but at least 25 percent of your fiber should be soluble (meaning it dissolves easily in water). Insoluble fiber helps you to have regular bowel movements and to clean your digestive system of toxins that might otherwise build up. A lot of diabetics suffer from poor bowel movements, irritable bowel syndrome, and frequent diarrhea because they're not getting enough fiber and what they are getting isn't easily absorbed by their body. This is a really important step for the rehabilitation of your body.

You can find insoluble fiber in whole-wheat products, corn, bran, grape, apple and pear skins, carrots, and in green vegetables like brussel sprouts, green beans, celery, and flaxseeds. Soluble fiber is found in rice, cereals, pasta, oatmeal, cornmeal, barley, quinoa, soy and papaya. Carrots, yams, sweet potatoes, turnips, pumpkins and mushrooms are also good sources and will help you feel full without spiking your blood sugar. Although you can always substitute with a fiber supplement, it is far better to get your fiber naturally and through these healthy sources. First, it's better for your body. Second, these health foods can help lower your bad LDL cholesterol and lower blood sugar levels.

At the same time, you're investing money in food rather than supplements. That's amazing and could be a life-changing (or life-saving) herbal treatment for Type 1 diabetics.

If you're following my recommendations, then the process of switching to the green drinks and then easing into these vitamin D and fiber regimens will have you about three months into your new lifestyle. At this point it's time to add a few additional natural supplements.

One of my favorites is aloe vera, the gel from the spiky green plant that you've probably used before for a sunburn or rash. Aloe vera is a great treatment though for other maladies, and it is one of the best natural colon cleansers (along with strong coffee). Although aloe vera contains a sugar, it doesn't have an adverse effect on blood sugar levels. In fact, the type of sugar found in aloe vera can actually help you overcome urinary tract infections, which are common in diabetics, particularly in women. Aloe vera is also a great source of protein, enzymes, calcium, selenium, magnesium, zinc, and the vitamins A and E. You'll also find amino acids and glutathione, that antioxidant we've discussed before.

Aloe vera is known to reduce blood sugar and triglycerides in many people. In fact, over the course of six weeks, many diabetics have seen a 40 percent reduction in their blood sugar and triglycerides when taking aloe vera. Since aloe vera juice has no taste, it's easy to add to a drink or recipe. Aloe vera has also been shown to reduce neuropathic pain, improve circulation, aid in wound healing, reduce the need for kidney dialysis, and even help regulate cholesterol levels.

Part of what is so great about this supplement is you can undoubtedly purchase and grow your own aloe vera plants! If not, you can still purchase the leaves at a grocery store. Of course, there are also all sorts of bottled aloe vera gels and dried oral supplements. You might want to include fresh aloe leaves or one of these concentrates in your green drinks first thing in the morning and get it all over at once!

I mentioned curcumin earlier, and it is widely accepted as an anti-inflammatory compound that is good in treatment of neurodegenerative, cardiovascular, pulmonary, metabolic, and autoimmune diseases. That's quite a list, isn't it! Additionally, in

Off the Grid with Diabetes

lab trials curcumin has been shown to reduce pain and insulin sensitivity while increasing glucose tolerance. It helps relieve painful neuropathies, protects memory, increases levels of glutathione, may help treat the effects of Alzheimer's disease (remember our reference to Type 3 diabetes), and of course it is all-natural!

In addition to cooking with turmeric spices whenever possible, you can also take curcumin as an extract. It is often listed as curcuma longa or turmeric extract. You might want to start at 1,000 milligrams a day (usually in two doses of 500 mg.) However, curcumin is often times poorly absorbed by the body, so you might want to consider taking black pepper along with curcumin. There are some high-quality supplements available in a special form, but again I want to encourage you to seek curcumin in the natural form whenever possible.

Fenugreek is another one we've already touched on briefly, and while you can cook with it, it is also valuable as a supplement. It helps promote healthy blood sugar levels and cholesterol in addition to being a strong antioxidant. Fenugreek lowers your free radical levels, meaning it could be effective against cancer cells, and it may help prevent varicose veins because the bioflavonoid rutin improves the strength of capillaries and veins. Scientists believe it helps prevent against metabolic syndrome by regulating blood pressure, blood sugar disorders, and high cholesterol.

Fenugreek is a commonly eaten food, but the seeds can be bitter and difficult to incorporate into recipes, making this an ideal supplement. If you take a capsule supplement, you can safely start at 1200 mg or so twice a day. However, fenugreek is something you can grow easily at home. You plant it in late spring, and it is ready to use in just a few months. You can also sprout the seeds and use them in salads to add a spicy flavor, or you can soak them in a glass of water over night, then remove them from the water and drink it.

Off the Grid with Diabetes

One of the great things about fenugreek is that not only is it great for treating diabetes and it can be used both in food or as a supplement, it is also a source of fiber and can be grown in your garden. You can probably tell I'm sold on fenugreek, and I hope you'll include it in your survival garden plans as well as your storage.

Another great herb I want to mention is gymnema sylvestre. This plant is native to India and has been used there for more than 2,000 years and is called the sugar destroyer for its effectiveness in treating diabetes. As a dietary supplement, it doesn't require a prescription, but it is still a powerful herb for lowering blood sugar. Since one of the side effects of gymnema is neutralizing the sweet taste of sugar in your mouth, it can help to suppress sugar cravings naturally.

This herb is so powerful that among Type 1 diabetics, nearly 100 percent of trial participants saw improvements in their insulin requirements, blood glucose levels, ATC counts, plasma proteins, and serum lipids after a year of supplementing with a water soluble extract of the leaves of gymnema sylvestre. That's amazing and could be a life changing (or life saving) herbal treatment for your child! Even better, there were no adverse side effects reported either, so no one should ever find themselves consigned to a life of insulin shots!

A good dosage would be 500mg twice a day of high quality gymnema sylvestre, if you're using it in capsule format. If you can get the leaves or powder, even better. As with all supplements, do your research on the quality and origin of the products you're buying.

Another natural gift from the east is ocimum sanctum, or holy basil. This is another one from India, but it can be grown right in your back yard. Holy basil helps improve the functioning of the beta cells in your pancreas, which we know is critical to proper insulin health. In fact, clinical trials have shown a 34

Off the Grid with Diabetes

percent decrease in fasting blood sugar levels after just a month of supplementing with holy basil leaves (or powder from the leaves)! Still better than drug results, and all natural!

Holy basil leaves have many advantages. They can have an antidepressant role in your brain and they are anti-inflammatory, which may help relieve arthritis. They are also antioxidants, may protect the heart against damage from cancer drugs, have been proven to help with metabolic syndrome, and can even help with heartburn and bloating. You can grow holy basil leaves and use them as a food or dry, crush, and grind them to use as a supplement (some people use 2.5 grams of dried leaf powder per day), or you can look for high-quality supplements from the holy basil leaf.

Lipoic acid is a fatty acid that occurs naturally in the body and is necessary for the production of energy and the conversion of glucose. Supplements that contain lipoic acid are therefore a good start on the reduction of blood sugar. However, it is tough to find good reliable sources of lipoic acid because so much of it is manufactured and therefore of suspect quality. However, generally speaking, when you find lipoic acid in your supplements, that's a good thing.

I also want to mention resveratrol, which is a powerful antioxidant found in cacao, red grapes, berries, and red wine. Resveratrol is a chemical released naturally in plants and has had remarkable results in lab tests. Studies have shown that even those with high-fat diets were able to attain normal life spans while avoiding heart disease and diabetes by supplementing with resveratrol. Other trials have shown that resveratrol has anti-cancer effects by suppressing the growth of cancer cells. The same anti-inflammatory effects make it great for combating the organ failure that often accompanies diabetes. Resveratrol improves thyroid function, helps to balance the good and bad cholesterol, reduces your risk for heart attack and stroke, protects your eyes from glaucoma, and simultaneously lowers your blood sugar levels.

However, many sources of resveratrol have very low absorption rates, with as much as 75 percent passing through your body unabsorbed. Finding higher-quality brands or liquid forms is therefore a real plus with this supplement. The root extract of polygonum cuspidatum is the scientific name, while it is sometimes known by the Chinese herbal name hu zhang.

When you're shopping for resveratrol, the higher the number on the supplement, the better. Resveratrol 50 has a 50 percent concentration of resveratrol, while 70 stands for 70 percent. Some products use fillers, which you want to avoid because they can cause diarrhea. Do some research to find a high-quality product with lots of good feedback before making a commitment.

This wraps up my review of the supplements that should form the basis of your new lifestyle. As you can see, the cause is not hopeless, and the disease is eminently treatable using natural herbs and minerals. You can treat the disease using off-grid, time-tested methods. However, as with anything else, a little preparation now will go a long way, and having a garden producing the fruits, vegetables, spices, and herbs you need is a lot better than trying to fill your pantry up with supplements, so don't waste a day! Get started right now!

Chapter Seven:

Off-Grid Exercising

Half the battle against diabetes in the long run is an active life that purges the body, burns fat, and maintains healthy cardiovascular and pulmonary health. Exercise also helps to offset those foods we may consume that are not ideal for our bodies, and in an off-grid environment, we won't be as selective about what we eat as we might be when we can go to a health food store.

Some survivalists maintain that in an off-grid environment we won't be eating enough to have diabetic problems, but this misses the point. If you've stocked your pantry with lots of highly processed, preserved foods, you will be consuming the worst possible diet imaginable for your health. Even if your caloric intake drops, the stress on your body will still be extraordinary!

Additionally, exercise has been proven to be a great antidote to stress, reducing the harmful hormones that sometimes are coursing through our bodies as we cope with "fight or flight" reactions to the environment around us, and a survival situation will undoubtedly be a stressful one for us. In short, our bodies are designed to be active, and if our work does not accomplish this, we need to add it back into our lifestyle to ensure proper balance.

I have devised a very simple but effective workout that you can do virtually anywhere and without any special equipment. In fact, this is part of the very same routine I used to lose 100 pounds and defeat diabetes. I did it without any special workout equipment, so I know it works!

This routine is based around a three-day-a-week workout schedule. I chose three days a week because I knew that I could commit an hour a day three times a week. You won't find

---

Off the Grid with Diabetes

yourself working out on back-to-back days where you're still sore from the previous day, and yet you'll be working out enough to be meaningful. Of course, this routine is just an idea, you can modify it in any way, but I began heavily overweight and out of shape and without any equipment. I've designed it with that in mind, so that you can learn a routine that you can take with you anywhere and maintain even under the worst circumstances.

Each day's routine will include some cardio activity to get your heart pumping and make you sweat as well as some muscle-training exercises. As your muscles grow, they eat all the time, burning sugar and reducing the stress on your system. This is why muscle development is so important. But we need both. You need to be able to walk around the block, over the hill, or away from danger! So let's get started!

Day 1

I recommend beginning each day's exercises with your cardio. This gets the blood flowing and warms up your whole body. You don't want to do the muscle exercises before the cardio because you might begin cramping. On that note, make sure you drink plenty of water before, during, and after you workout. If you find yourself thirsty in the evening after your workout, make sure you drink lots of water and avoid coffee and alcohol. Thirst is a sign that your body is already dehydrated!

On this day I recommend beginning with a walk. The walk should be vigorous, not the lazy kind of loitering teens do at the mall, but the active kind that you see the old mall walkers doing, like they're hurrying to get to the ice cream shop for a free scoop! You should be walking fast enough that it's a real effort. You can walk around a track, around the neighborhood, indoors, or cross-country.

Off the Grid with Diabetes

Whatever kind of walking you do, make sure you have great shoes. They should be quality walking shoes, they should fit you well, and they should be comfortable. If you're going to walk cross-country, make sure you have proper ankle support and that you use extra caution to avoid hidden risks to foot and ankle health, like debris or holes in the earth. I recommend you walk for about twenty minutes. At a good pace, you should easily get a mile done in this time. It is a good idea to mark off a mile in your vehicle so you have some idea of the distance. The mile isn't particularly important, whether it's a little less or a little more, but unless you have an injury, this is a good measurement of the proper pace.

After you've finished the twenty minutes (or so) of walking, and while you're still warm and your heart rate is up, I recommend either working on the stairs or doing a similar exercise. Here's what I mean by stairs: if you've got stairs in your home or at a public place, I want you to ascend the stairs as quickly as possible. That's not necessarily running, but faster than you might normally. Think of going up the steps like an eager child. Don't skip any steps; make sure you hit every one.

There are several ways to approach the steps. You can hit each step alternating between left and right foot on alternate steps, or you can hit each step with both feet. This will feel slightly uncomfortable at first, but you'll also find out how much of a workout it really is! Regardless of how you do it, when you arrive at the top of the steps, immediately reverse course and come back down. Don't run—just walk down the stairs, and then begin all over again. The idea is to ascend as quickly as possible, walk down, and then do it again. Your heart will be pumping like crazy! Set a goal for yourself—maybe five cycles of up/down, then increase it to seven, then ten, then fifteen, and so forth. Your current level of conditioning will determine all this. You must push yourself though, until you're sweating and out of breath.

If you don't have access to stairs, you can do a modified version of this on a bench, or even on the front step to your home, a curb, a rock, a tree stump, or any elevated step. Take a step up, bring your second foot up alongside the first, and then return to the ground. Repeat, always starting with the same foot. After doing twenty of these, switch it up and begin with the other foot. You'll find yourself getting pretty winded. Just be careful that the step up isn't too high for you or you risk pulling a muscle.

The final cardio exercise for the day is jumping jacks. You probably haven't done these in years, but after a few awkward moments you'll have the rhythm back again. Just remember that as your feet come together at the bottom of the move, your hands should come to the side of your legs. Conversely, when your legs are apart your arms should be up in the 'Y' form. I would suggest starting with twenty-five of these (unless you can do fifty), and you should do three sets of these separated by sixty seconds of resting.

With this complete, your cardio for the day is over, and you should proceed immediately to the muscle workout. It's critical that you move into this right away and don't cool down, so that you get the maximum out of your workout.

Each day's workout has a circuit of sorts to follow, although the order is not particularly important. I tend to work the larger muscles first, but it's not that important. In the Day 1 routine, I like to start with squats, since we just came off a leg-intensive routine. This really puts the muscle group under stress. That's a good thing when you're trying to build muscle mass!

Squats are simple exercises. Plant your feet about shoulder width apart, fold your arms across your chest, and then simply squat down, so that your upper legs are parallel to the floor. Do NOT squat all the way down so that your rear is on your heels! You are likely to injure yourself that way! Just come down to approximately halfway, and then return to the normal standing position. Most people can do twenty of these without too much difficulty. It should be tough, but not impossible. Wait thirty seconds, and then do another set. Wait another thirty seconds, and then do a third and final set. If you can do twenty-five, thirty, or thirty-five of each set, then great! What you want to be able to do is three sets of whatever amount, and when that third set at that level is easy to accomplish, you know you need to increase the number by five or more (per set).

Now we're going to move away from your legs (breathe a sigh of relief!), and work on your core. Your core muscles in the abdomen and back are key to your overall health and strength. The stronger you are here, the less strain you put on the back and the rest of your body. So, each day's workout will have a core component to it. Day 1's core workout is the crunch.

A crunch is the beginning of a sit-up, but the key difference is that in the crunch only the top part of your body (really just the shoulders) is raised up, and the rest of your back remains on the floor. This crunch exercise works the abdomen without putting a lot of strain on the lower back. I recommend that you put your arms out in front of you at a 45-degree angle, and as you crunch inwards towards your bent knees, pretend like you're trying to touch a ball that is suspended over your knees. If you assume the proper position, you will find that your abs are under constant stress, and that's what we want! Some people can do ten, fifteen, or twenty of these crunches without a problem, but when I first started all I could do was ten. Whatever the number, make sure you maintain good posture, and do them correctly. If you can only do ten, then do the ten, count to thirty, and then do your second set. Wait another thirty seconds, and then do a third set.

Next on our Day 1 workout is the shoulder muscles. These are critical for lifting and holding tools, carrying things, and moving things. If you've not been working out much, you might find that these muscles are really weak. On the other hand, I have found that mothers of young children are strong in the shoulders from all the lifting of little ones!

This is an exercise that requires some weights. No, not weights you have to buy at the gym, but just a little extra resistance. It might be a water bottle, a book, a milk jug, or even a rock. I began with a water bottle, full of water. After a few weeks I replaced the water with sand. Then I added water to the sand. Eventually I moved from that little water bottle to a gallon milk jug! These kinds of weights are handy, inexpensive, and just as effective as store-bought weights.

Next we are going to be working your deltoids. The first exercise involves holding the bottle in your hand and, while keeping your arm stiff and straight, lifting the bottle in front of you until it is level with your shoulder, then returning it to your side. You can alternate arms this way (if you have two bottles), or you can do them all on one arm and then switch.

After you have done a set in front, we're now going to work the sides. Holding the bottle directly in front of your abdomen, swing the bottle out to your side, like you are forming a cross. Again, bring the bottle up to shoulder level while keeping your arm straight and stiff. Do this ten or fifteen times. I bet your shoulders will be burning! That's okay. Take a thirty-second break and then repeat these exercises a second and third time. I know, it hurts, but that means good stuff is happening.

Next up on Day 1 is a return to the legs and core exercise. Lie down on the floor, flat on your back. Put your hands under your butt, with your palms on the floor. What we're doing is the scissor exercise. You will be raising your feet together, just a few inches, and then spreading them, like scissors. So, with feet together, on the floor, lift up, then spread them out, bring them back together and then back down to the floor. That's one! Repeat at least ten times; do fifteen if you can. I like to keep my head on the floor, but some people like to keep their head up (chin to chest). I always feel like that puts too much stress on my neck. So, keep your head back and focus on your lower abs and leg workout. Do those scissors slowly and methodically. When you've done the set, count to thirty, and then do the second and third set.

Since you're already down there, let's do some toe kicks. While in the same position, you're going to be raising your feet off the ground independent of one another, but only a few inches each, like you're kicking at something that's maybe a foot off the ground. Imagine you're shuffling in the air, and do this twenty times or so. Then stop, take a break, and repeat. When you've done these three sets, you're finished with core and legs!

The next Day 1 exercise is the butterfly. Grab those bottles you were using for the deltoid exercise, lie flat on your back, arms extended in a cross formation, and with a bottle in each hand, keep your arms straight and bring them up directly over your breast, in slow motion. You're working your pectoral muscles this way. If you can do fifteen of these, great! Do three sets as with the other exercises.

We're almost done! Since your bottles are still handy, let's do some shrugs. This might require a heavier bottle than what you were using for some of your other exercises. If you were using little water bottles for your earlier exercises, you might want a larger bottle or something filled with sand instead of water. Anyway, these exercises are very easy . . . holding one bottle in each hand, simply shrug your shoulders. There are several ways to do this. You can pinch your shoulders up directly against your neck, or you can roll them forward and backwards. I suggest all three! You ought to be able to do a lot of reps of these— your shoulders are really strong, so do fifteen or twenty shrugs each way. The tendency with this exercise is to unconsciously lift the bottles with your arms, so try to resist that by keeping your arms straight, and in your mind visualize working your shoulders in this way. Just thinking about the proper form really helps!

When you're done with the three sets of shrugs, you're on to your last exercise! We're going to wrap up with one more shoulder exercise. Sitting in a chair or on a bench and using those trusty bottles from before, lift them straight up into the air, directly over your shoulders, just like you're stretching. Keep your back nice and straight

Off the Grid with Diabetes

and push those bottles into the air. If you can do fifteen, great! Do this fifteen times, and do three sets. If fifteen is easy, you need to use a heavier bottle.

You're done with the Day 1 exercises! Congratulations!

Day 2

What I call Day 2 is the second of your three-day workout, but I recommend that it be separated by one day from workout Day 1. You might workout Monday, Wednesday, and Friday or Tuesday, Thursday and Saturday to keep a regular balance and have enough rest as well.

On Day 2, you'll begin again with cardio, starting first with walking. If you walked on a track or a sidewalk on Day 1, it would be a good idea to change things up. Try walking up and down some hills, or through the woods, or around your property. Diversity in your workout is a good thing so your muscles are constantly being stressed and challenged. It may not seem like it, but just walking around your property gives you a very different workout than say, walking laps at the track. Walking around the mall is different from walking hills in your neighborhood. Your stride is different, your pace is different, and even how your foot impacts the ground is different. Of course, I suggest you walk outside whenever possible and on a natural surface rather than concrete or asphalt. It's easier on your body that way. I think the diversity helps you psychologically as well, when you think to yourself, "Oh, today I'm going to walk _____," rather than thinking, "Oh, another day of walking."

So walk for twenty minutes or so, get a mile in, then I want you to begin running in place. Running in place really elevates your heart rate, so it is great exercise, but you vastly lower your risk of injury compared to true jogging. Plus, you can do it virtually anywhere. At first, if you are out of shape, you may find that even sixty seconds of jogging in place is difficult, so just pace yourself. If you can only do thirty seconds, do that, rest, and then do another thirty seconds. The goal is that you would be able to get up to five minutes running in place. Take it one step at a time.

The final portion of your cardio on Day 2 is jump rope. A little like jumping jacks, you may not have done these in a long time, but they're a great exercise. It doesn't matter if you don't have a true jump rope, just grab any rope and cut it to the right length. If you've not done jump rope in awhile, it might be a little awkward. Take it easy; just work on getting the timing down right and your own movements. You should focus on twirling the rope in your fingers, not a lot of arm motion, and your jumps should really resemble more like bunny hops than jumps. Don't let your knees bend more than necessary to cushion the up and down motion, and propel yourself up just enough to let that rope under your feet. Often I see people who aren't moving the rope fast enough. It takes some practice, but in no time you'll be jumping away!

Start off trying to do twenty-five at a time. You should be able to do three sets of twenty-five. Eventually I want you to work up to fifty at least three times. You may find that once you've developed a routine, doing fifty is nothing, so of course, adjust upwards as you need to in order to challenge yourself. Work your way up to 75 and then 100 without stopping!

Off the Grid with Diabetes

Now that you're done with cardio, it's time to move on to the muscle workout for Day 2. We'll begin today by working the thighs. Find a wall and put your back to it. Position your feet in front of you slightly, then slide down the wall and mimic the position of sitting in a chair. Your back should be flat to the wall and your upper legs should be parallel to the floor. Keep your arms either across your chest or out in front of you. The temptation will be to put your hands on your thighs or knees, so keep them away. Try to hold that position for thirty seconds on your first try. If you've not done much exercising, you might find this difficult. But make that your first goal, and do three repetitions at thirty seconds each, and as you can, gradually increase it to forty-five seconds, then sixty seconds. You'll be there in no time!

The next exercise is designed to improve your calf strength. With stronger calf muscles you can walk and run easier, go up stairs, even pick things up with less strain on your back. With the calf raise, you are simply going to lift your body weight by pushing yourself from a flat-footed standing position up onto your tip toes. For most people, to do this fifteen or twenty times on both feet isn't much of a challenge. So, what I recommend is to lift one leg, exercising only one leg at a time. It will help to use a wall or doorframe as balance. So, let's assume you are working your right calf, then put your left arm out to brace yourself against a doorframe or wall. Resist the urge to lean into the wall, making the exercise easier. Just use it to help with your balance as you push up onto your tiptoes. Do fifteen to twenty of these, then switch to the other leg and repeat. When you can do fifteen calf raises three times, begin shooting for twenty. Once you can do twenty, then begin doing the exercise holding a milk jug full of water or sand in the hand on the same side as the calf you're working.

There are several ways to change this exercise in order to work a slightly different set of muscles: for example, you can turn your foot in or out slightly and you'll notice a difference in the difficulty of the exercise. You can also place a board, carpet, or any other item under the ball of your foot, allowing your heel to drop down slightly lower. When you rise up, you'll find the movement more difficult, because you're on an incline. Before long, you'll have weight on your hand and a board under your feet and calves that look like a long jumper's!

Once you've given those calves a workout, let's switch things up and do some core workouts. One of my favorites is the plank. Some of the reasons I like it so much are that anyone can do it anywhere, it works so many muscles, and I haven't figured out a way to hurt yourself doing it.

Here's how it works: lie face down on the carpet, resting on your elbows. Your elbows should be approximately shoulder-width apart, with your hands clasped in front of you. What you are going to do is elevate your entire body off the ground, so that only your elbows and toes are touching the ground. You should resemble a plank of wood from shoulders to heels. You should not have your butt sticking up in the air making an inverted V, nor should you be sagging in the middle. You should be perfectly straight and then hold this position. Initially you may only be able to do a thirty-second plank before the shaking and exhaustion takes over. That's okay! Do that three times and begin to work your way up to forty-five seconds and then sixty seconds three times! This exercise builds everything from your shoulders through your core to your butt muscles and your legs. You'll get so much strength from this exercise; you'll notice it almost immediately in your daily life. Plus, you don't risk hurting yourself or pulling any muscles. Once you're done with the plank, you will probably want to rest. That's okay. Take a moment before starting the next exercise.

After a sixty-second rest, assume a prostrate position, arms out in front of you, palms down. This exercise is going to work your arms, back, shoulders, butt and legs. What you're going to do is raise your right arm and left leg up slightly and in conjunction together. You only need to lift them about six inches off the ground, then lower them. Do this fifteen to twenty times. Then switch to the other side and repeat. You'll do three sets of fifteen to twenty repetitions on each side. This is a great way exercise several different muscle groups!

Next, we're going to work your triceps. If you have a bottle you've been using, this is a great exercise for it. Grasp the bottle in your hand, bend your arm backwards over your shoulder, bottle behind your ear, and then lift it straight up, flexing your elbows so that you are using your triceps alone to power the push. Do this fifteen times and then switch hands. Repeat that process until you've done three sets. If you're not working with bottles or don't have one available, you can work this same muscle group using a chair or even a step. Turn your back to the chair, put your hands behind you on the edge of the chair, and then lower yourself about a foot. Your legs should be straight out in front of you, not supporting your weight. As you lower yourself down, resist the urge to use your thighs to hold you up. You want to lower yourself past the point where your thighs are parallel to the ground, because this is the point where your triceps are bearing the weight. Go slowly, because there is a point where your weight is shifted to your shoulders and not your triceps. That's a bad thing. So when you feel that begin to happen, stop and push yourself back up. Do three sets of fifteen of these.

The next exercise is a fundamental part of any workout: the pushup. This works your pectoral muscles as well as your arms. It's essential for upper body strength. The classic position of the cross shape, with legs extended but together, face down, and hands on the ground at shoulder length is perfect. Your head should be up, looking forward, rather than face down. You want to lower yourself slowly until your chest would touch a baseball on the floor, and then raise yourself slowly to the point where your arms are fully extended.

If you have trouble doing these pushups, there are a number of variations to help make the transition. I do not recommend pushups that keep your knees on the ground because it's so difficult to keep good form. Instead, if you can't do a pushup the normal way, then find something elevated to put your hands on. This might be a park bench, two chairs on either side of your chest, a couch, or the steps. By elevating your upper body, you're shifting your weight to your feet, meaning you don't have to lift as much weight.

You can also vary your hand position. The closer your hands are together, the more weight you're putting on your triceps, and the further apart they are, the more weight you are putting on your pecs. Change them up just to provide a challenge to your body. If you have trouble with your wrists, you can make a fist and put your fist down onto the ground instead of your palm. This is a

Off the Grid with Diabetes

harder pushup but spares your wrist. If you want a more challenging pushup, you can put your palms together in the diamond form directly below your chest, or put your feet up on something, like a step or chair, shifting more of the weight to your chest and mimicking a bench-press-type exercise. By the way, the normal style pushup utilizes about 65 percent of your body weight. If you fold your legs over one another (so only foot is on the ground), or elevate your feet, you're just increasing the difficulty. Constantly alternate these exercises to challenge yourself. Work your way up to three sets of twenty pushups.

The last exercise of the day is the butterfly. For this one you will lie on your back on the ground, or on a bench or bed, with your arms out to the side and a bottle in each hand. All you are going to do is bring the bottles together directly over your chest. Then slowly bring them back down. If you can lie on a bench, you can get your hands slightly below the level of your chest, and this gives you a little extra challenge, but even if you are just doing this on the floor you get a good workout. Do it slowly, maintaining good form, and when you lower the bottles, don't let your arms come to a complete rest on the ground—keep some weight on them at all times and you will find the exercise can be really challenging. Do fifteen of these three times, and guess what? You're done with Day 2!

Day 3

On Day 3 of this routine we will wrap up the cycle of exercises using modifications of the techniques we have employed in the previous days.

For cardio, we'll begin again with approximately one mile of walking. Try to vary your routine from Day 1 and Day 2 with a change in scenery, pace, or location. After approximately twenty minutes of vigorous walking, proceed to jump squats. A jump squat is just what it sounds like: you assume a squat position and extend your arms above your head as if to reach the sky, and then jump as high as you can. You will do three sets of these and fifteen repetitions each.

When you're done with the jump squats, we'll finish the cardio portion with sprints. An ideal wind sprint is a short distance run, followed by walking. Make sure you stretch your legs before sprinting. A good distance to sprint is thirty steps or about the length of a basketball court. Gradually increase to fifty steps, then seventy-five steps. A sprint is an all-out dash, not an easy jogging-type pace. Your heart should be pounding when you finish the sprint. Make sure you continue to walk between sprints, and they should be separated by no more than thirty-second rest periods. You should do six to ten sprints, gradually increasing the distance.

Once you finish the cardio, begin the strength exercises. The first is a variation of the squats we performed on Day 2. These squats are called sumo style because you place your legs farther apart than normal and your toes are pointed outward rather than directly forward. Put your arms across your chest, squat to parallel with the floor and then back up. At first, these will feel like regular squats, but after just a few you'll find that they are working a very different portion of your leg. The next day you'll really feel a difference. When you first begin, you might find that you can only do fifteen of these. Work your way up to twenty-five or thirty per set, and do three sets, separated by no more than a sixty-second pause.

Off the Grid with Diabetes

Now let's move to the core workout portion. Begin with reverse crunches. Lie on the floor and place your hands on the floor or behind your head. Bring your knees in towards your chest until they're bent to 90 degrees, with your feet together or crossed. Contract your abs to curl your hips off the floor, reaching your legs up toward the ceiling. Lower and repeat, doing three sets of ten to fifteen reps.

For the next exercise, remain on your back, legs extended, feet together. You'll need either a partner for these or an object to work against. For example, the first exercise is a lift, so you will hold your legs straight out in front of you, palms under your butt, lifting your feet a few inches off the ground while your partner pushes against them. They're not trying to push your legs to the floor, just providing resistance. If you don't have a partner you can put weight on your ankles or find something else to work against, like the underside of a chair, shelf, or step. Do three sets of these, counting to fifteen for each set.

Next is the leg push down. Assume the same position as with the lift, but you will be pushing down with your feet rather than pushing up. So, a partner here would be holding your heels while with legs together you push down. Try not to raise your butt off the ground. If you don't have a partner, you can push against a rock, a step, or anything that is elevated about six inches or so. Do three sets of fifteen seconds each.

The next resistance exercise is the horizontal push. You will have your feet together as before, but this time your partner will sit off to the side. If you are pushing to the right, he will be seated to your right. As you lift your legs up, he will hold your ankles against the side of his leg and you will push to the right. Your body will want to contort itself into a V, folding in the direction you're pushing, but resist that and try to maintain good form. Of course, if you don't have a partner, you can do this against any immobile object. Do three sets of fifteen seconds each. After you've pushed to the right, your partner will switch and position himself on your left side. Again, do three sets of fifteen seconds each.

Next, your partner will sit at the end of your feet and you will put your feet between his calves. Here you will be attempting to spread your legs apart. He will hold them together while for fifteen seconds you attempt to mimic the scissor spread from an earlier exercise. Do three sets.

Next, your partner will remain in this position but put your feet on the outside of his calves while you will attempt to close the scissors. Again, he will hold your heels up to the outside of his calves, and you will push in for fifteen seconds. As with before, do three sets.

The final core/leg workout involves turning over on your stomach and bending your knees. Your partner will hold the tops of your feet and you will attempt to push back against him. He will have to hold your feet or toes tightly, because your legs will be very strong compared to his upper body strength. Do three sets with fifteen seconds of resistance. Then reverse. With legs straight out, your partner will hold your heels while you try to raise them up to your butt. Again, do three sets for fifteen seconds each.

With all of these exercises you should work up your resistance time. Maybe you will have trouble with fifteen seconds at first, so only do ten. Maybe you can do twenty or twenty-five with just a little effort. Use a stopwatch to time your sessions, because you will naturally count faster as you reach the ends of the set. Also, if you don't have a partner, don't despair; you can find other objects to work against that will give you the resistance you need for each exercise.

Let's work the arms now. One of my favorite arm exercises can be performed with just a few simple objects. Tie a rope that is about five feet long around the middle of a stick or a broken mop or broom handle. Then tie a weight to the other end of the rope. Hold the stick out in front of you at chest level (your arms should be level), and then proceed to roll up the rope by twisting the stick away from you. Go slowly—emphasize your right arm, then your left arm as you reel that weight up to the top of the stick. Then reverse course and slowly lower the weight again. That's one set. For the next set, you might want to alternate, holding the stick with your palms up instead of down. This works a different part of your arm and will put less stress on your fingers. It may be a little more awkward to do, but it's a great variation. For the third set, you might want to reel the rope up in the opposite direction. This will really work those muscles, and whether you're a homemaker or desk jockey, you'll suddenly find more strength in everything you do.

Next is the simple bicep curl. There are lots of ways to do this, and I want you to alternate as you do each set. Take one of your bottles, and standing, hold the bottle right to your hip, then lift slowly until your forearm comes close to the bicep or 'closes' completely. Lift slowly and return slowly. Make sure you are not using your upper body to help you with this bicep curl. After you've done twelve to fifteen, switch arms. I like to actually put the arm that isn't working over my bicep to help keep good form. After the first set, you might want to try this exercise sitting on the corner of a chair or bed, or even at the stairs, where you can spread your legs and do the curl inside the thigh of whatever arm you're working. So, if you're doing the right bicep, put your arm on the inside of your right thigh. Lean over so that you can complete the curl inside your legs. Another variation on the curl is to hold the bottle or weight differently. Instead of palm up, turn your palm inward, like you are about to shake hands, and then curl the weight toward you. This is called a hammer in weight-lifting circles. You can do this sitting, standing, or in the leaning-over preacher curl.

Next we'll do a modified bench press. Lie on your back with a weight in each hand. Start with the weights at your chest and push directly up until your arms are fully extended. Then slowly bring them back down to your chest. For a modification, you can do this close in, so your hands are almost together, or alternate so they are further apart. The further apart they are, the more you are working your chest. Do three sets of fifteen reps.

The final exercise of the routine is a shoulder press. Sitting upright in a chair, begin with your bottles in each hand at shoulder level and push them straight up and return. Do these slowly, and do fifteen repetitions per set.

Congratulations, you're finished! If you incorporate this routine into your life three days a week, as I have suggested, you can achieve physical health and strength, endurance, and vitality. You don't have to invest in fancy health equipment or a gym membership that you won't use or may not have access to. In an off-grid situation, you're going to need your strength and endurance. For those who are suffering from diabetes, building

Off the Grid with Diabetes

up the extra muscle mass gives you an offensive weapon against the buildup of excess sugar in your system. Those muscles are burning sugar around the clock, and the more sugar they burn, the less excess there is in your body. The bigger the muscle and the more often you use it, the more sugar it will burn. Before you know it, not only will your muscles be burning the excess sugar in your system, but also they will be burning up that extra fat you've got around your midsection, thighs, and buttocks!

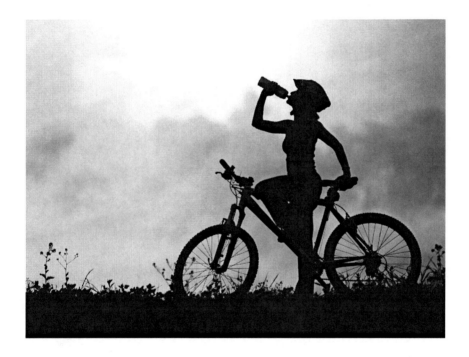

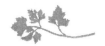

Chapter Eight:

Solutions Targeted to Common Diabetic Concerns

Sometimes the diabetic disease goes undiagnosed for a long time and the damage to organs and tissue manifests itself before it is possible to reverse the consequences. Other times, even when blood sugar is brought under control, organs are sufficiently weakened that they succumb to failure or infection. This can be a frustrating problem.

Of course, in an off-grid situation, problems may develop that under normal circumstances might have been identified in a medical environment, but go unnoticed until it is too late to bring about preventive care. In this chapter, I'll address some of the more common problems diabetics face and the steps you can take to mitigate against them.

One of the most common and serious complications of diabetes is vision loss or deteriorating vision. People with diabetes are twice as likely to develop cataracts or glaucoma as are the normal population. In fact, diabetics make up 8 percent of all those considered legally blind, and diabetics make up a significant percentage of all new cases of blindness in adults between the ages of 20 and 74. More alarming, about 20 percent of all newly diagnosed diabetics already have some form of retinopathy. It's a very serious threat to anyone, but particularly in an off-grid lifestyle because the laser surgeries that might otherwise help in a normal situation won't be available.

First, let's review some of the most common eye problems confronting diabetics, so you can be aware of the risks that you or any diabetic will face. Diabetic retinopathy is a condition that

---

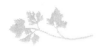

causes blurred vision, floaters, flashes of light, or even total loss of vision when blood vessels in the retina weaken and then leak. This leakage causes pressure on the part of the retina that is responsible for clear vision. The longer you have high blood sugar, the greater the risk of this condition and the worse it is likely to become.

Macular degeneration is the loss of the central portion of your vision. Typical symptoms of macular degeneration are blurred lines in your vision, fading colors, and wavy lines of distortion. It is most common among the elderly but also among untreated diabetics.

Floaters are those tiny spots or squiggly lines that drift into your field of vision, especially if you look at something bright such as white paper or a clear blue sky. Most of the time these are benign and no cause to worry. However, if your floaters are accompanied by flashes of light or a loss of peripheral vision, then it may be a more serious side effect of diabetic retinopathy and of course, more difficult to treat.

When cloudiness begins to manifest in the lens of the eye, we call it a cataract. With that cloud obscuring your vision, things will appear blurry; you will become sensitive to light, see halos, and likely have very poor night vision.

When pressure in the eye begins to build up from fluid that is retained or not dealt with properly, the result can be poor night vision, a loss of peripheral vision, blind spots, and even total blindness. This is the glaucoma we mentioned earlier.

Presbyopia is the medical term for aging eyes. What happens is the lens of the eye loses its flexibility and isn't able to focus properly on items that are near.

If the optic nerve is inflamed, it is known as optic neuritis. A sign of optic neuritis is pain when you move your eyes from left to right. Colors may become faded and vision loss may accompany this pain. If you have a terrible pain in your eye, this may be ophthalmic migraines, which are a sort of spasm in your eye. The blood vessel behind your eye may respond to stress, poor diet, or neurological problems and produce these results.

Some basic discussion of good preventive care might be in order here. Always shade your eyes from the damage of the ultraviolet damage that is possible from UV rays. Good quality sunglasses are a wise investment, especially if you spend a lot of time in the sun (as you might in an off-grid situation). Of course, you'll want to guard your eyes from physical damage. Eye protection may not be sexy, but chemicals, dust, and smoke can cause serious problems. If you spend a lot of time reading, writing, watching TV, or using the computer, you might want to make sure to take regular breaks and rest your eyes, or even invest in a lubricating eye solution to aid healing. You can overuse your eyes, especially if they are engaged in a lot of intensive focusing.

One of the simplest behaviors to ensure eye health is frequent washing of your hands. If you are constantly touching your eyes (and most of us do, even if we don't realize it), then you may be bringing them into contact with germs that can be harmful. Another easy step towards eye health is to stop smoking. The smoke is terrible for your eyes because free radicals can damage sensitive eye capillaries.

Finally, I must encourage you to get a good amount of quality sleep. If you don't rest your eyes, they are like any other muscle or organ that is overtaxed; they begin to deteriorate and malfunction. You will notice the first signs of fatigue in your eyes, which is why the philosophers have always called the eyes the windows to the soul. Puffy eyes, bloodshot eyes, dark circles, or twitching in the eyes indicate both that the eyes are under strain and that there is almost certainly another underlying problem.

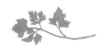

More worrying, there are some medications that are known to adversely affect your vision, including antihistamines, cold medicines, psychiatric medications, medication for urinary incontinence, and a long list of other chemicals. Research any medicine you're taking and see if it is linked to eye problems. Remember, manufacturers are in the business of selling drugs, not informing a small group of diabetics who are already at risk of eye problems that their drug may be dangerous.

Let's revisit some of the common problems we've already discussed and look at some of the treatments. Glaucoma should top our list both because of the prevalence and seriousness of the condition. One of the natural treatments that always tops the list when discussing glaucoma is marijuana, so let's discuss that first. Since 1992 there has been evidence that marijuana, taken orally or through inhalation, can lower intraocular pressure. For this reason, it is legal in some states with a prescription. Others caution that while it has been proven to lower intraocular pressure, the difference is not substantial. At the same time, the side effects of marijuana include drowsiness and hunger pangs. I believe these side effects more than offset the potential benefits from marijuana use.

Fortunately, there are a great many nutrients that are legal, safe, and widely available. Not only can they protect your eyesight, but they can also help to reverse damage done by this disease. At the top of our list is lutein, a yellow-orange pigment that is responsible for the color in many fruits and vegetables and is also an antioxidant with a proven impact on eye health. Lutein has also been shown to help prevent cataracts and macular degeneration. Unfortunately, humans cannot synthesize this nutrient, only plants can, so we have to get lutein from a plant-based food or a supplement.

While there are no RDA suggestions for lutein, most medical professionals say that we need six to ten milligrams a day to maintain eye health. You can get twice this amount in a one-cup serving of spinach or kale. In fact, excellent sources for lutein are any dark green leafy vegetables, including kale, spinach, Swiss chard, mustard greens, red leaf lettuce, parsley, and broccoli. Still rich in lutein but further down my preference list are tomatoes, corn, eggs, avocados, sweet potatoes, squash, mangoes, and papaya. Including these foods in your diet will help with your natural intake of lutein. If you can't make these foods prevalent enough in your diet or if you want an extra boost of lutein, you can find supplements easily, which should always be taken with a meal.

Another colorful pigment, similar to lutein and just as beneficial to the eye is zeaxanthin. Zeaxanthin quenches free radicals and prevents damage to the retina. We cannot make zeaxanthin, so we need to eat raw spinach leaves, broccoli, corn, and persimmons to get the highest concentration of this nutrient possible. The second tier foods include Brussels sprouts, peas, cauliflower, kale, and egg yolks. Of course, you can also find zeaxanthin in supplement form, and you may even find it in combination with lutein. A typical dose would be 4 milligrams daily.

Another carotenoid that is great for your eye health is beta-carotene. It gives carrots and pumpkins their color and is also the pigment we see in beautiful autumn leaves. When chlorophyll dies, it is the beta-carotene that we see. Beta-carotene can also undergo a transformation in the body and convert to a vitamin A called retinol.

There are some critics of retinol and beta-carotene, but they generally seem to have concerns about synthetic, manufactured beta-carotene. We already know why that kind of synthetic can be harmful. But natural, real beta-carotene has repeatedly been shown to protect your eyesight and is also a powerful antioxidant that may also help fight against cancer. Since people with vision problems are almost always deficient in vitamin A, beta-

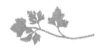

carotene can be a great supplement. Make sure you find only natural forms of beta-carotene, and I suggest those products that are from an algae or palm source.

You'll find beta-carotene naturally in sweet potatoes, butternut squash, tomatoes, spinach, cantaloupe, peaches, carrots, red peppers, pumpkin, collards, apricots, and broccoli. If you steam or sauté these veggies, you may find it even easier to absorb the beta-carotene. Great sources of vitamin A directly are meat, liver, kidney, butter, and eggs.

Another colorful, natural friend of the eye is the bilberry. This is a relative of the American blueberry, and it is actually blue in the center of the fruit, where the meat is. Bilberries contain a lot of vitamin C. They're also a great source of anthocyanosides, which are antioxidants and give the bilberry its strength in combating cataracts, macular degeneration, and glaucoma. In Europe they are in love with this natural treatment and trace the origins to pilots who would eat bilberry jam and find that they could see better in the dark! Not only do bilberries have a proven impact on night vision, but they can also lower blood sugar, reduce inflammatory chemicals, improve floaters, protect the retina, and strengthen capillary walls.

You might find that growing the bilberry is difficult or impossible (or just impractical), but you can find bilberry supplements in most health food stores. Make sure that the supplement you choose has 25 percent anthocyanosides, meaning that the supplement contains the most beneficial active ingredients.

Another great herb with a lot of promise is the gingko biloba herb that studies have shown has a beneficial effect on the optic nerve. Because so many people with diabetes have circulation problems that can impact the blood vessels leading to the eye, ginkgo can be helpful by thinning the blood and improving circulation. In past clinical tests, those diabetics who used ginkgo for a few months found fewer incidents of blood clotting and retinal blood flow was improved. More blood flow means more oxygen to the optic nerve and retina, meaning better eyesight. You can get ginkgo biloba tea or take 40 milligrams of ginkgo daily with food. Do not combine ginkgo with aspirin, heparin, warfarin, or any blood thinners because of its powerful combination effects.

Vitamin B is also great for your eyes and has a proven link for lower risk of macular degeneration. In a study that lasted seven years, women who took a B vitamin cocktail that also included folic acid had a 34 percent lower risk of macular degeneration and a 41 percent lower risk of significant visual impairment. You already know the many other healthy benefits of vitamin B, so you will want to maximize this in your diet. The great thing is that many of the green leafy vegetables I've already recommended are good sources of this, including broccoli, lettuce, parsley, turnip greens, Swiss chard, and kale. If you can't get the vitamin B naturally, you can find a high-quality B complex supplement.

Finally, studies have shown that omega-3 fatty acids can be helpful for immune system, blood flow, inflammation, and overall eye health. You can get omega-3 fatty acids from wild, cold-water fish such as Arctic char, salmon, cod, herring, anchovies, mackerel, and yellow fin or ahi tuna. You can also find many quality omega-3 fatty acid supplements that contain fish oil and krill oil. Krill oil is the best because it causes fewer abdominal discomforts. As always, do your research on the product and manufacturer.

Diabetics are not just at greater risk for eye problems, but also heart problems. We already know that one in three Americans have some type of cardiovascular disease. Half of those are over sixty. Many of the rest are already diabetic. One in four Americans has high blood pressure, and one in ten with cardiovascular disease have already had a heart attack. Nearly a quarter of all annual deaths in our country are linked to heart disease. It's the number one killer of Americans!

# Off the Grid with Diabetes

Diabetics are at a very high risk of developing heart disease, just compounding the problems diabetics already face. If you have high blood pressure, high cholesterol, or weight that is considered obese, you have the characteristics of someone who will develop heart disease. If you smoke or live a sedentary life, you've just bumped your risk even further.

A few symptoms you should learn and associate with heart problems include a sensation of pressure or squeezing in your chest, neck, or the top of your abdomen; irregular or fluttering heartbeat; lightheadedness or dizziness; the desire to sleep during the day; or shortness of breath. All these might be symptoms of a heart-related problem. Given the seriousness of this problem, let's talk about the supplements that can help prevent heart problems.

Among the best heart healthy supplements is arginine, an amino acid that is naturally occurring in your body, particularly in your pituitary gland. Arginine is tied to healthy blood sugar and blood pressure and can also boost energy levels. It helps to clear your arteries, lower cholesterol levels, and support your kidneys. It can also enhance healing and even support blood flow to sexual organs. Sound like a miracle drug? This amino acid really is a naturally occurring miracle! Rich sources of arginine in your diet are brown rice, coconut, oatmeal, seeds, whole-wheat bread, raisins, and nuts. You'll find lower levels of arginine in poultry and red meat.

I can't recommend artificial sources of arginine for several reasons, the most important of which is that side effects include blood thinning, stomach discomfort, bloating, and diarrhea. This is why I would highly recommend you utilize natural sources in your diet to correct deficiencies.

Another great heart healthy supplement is the vitamin-like coenzyme Q10. It's a powerful antioxidant and is found in the mitochondria of your cells. COQ10 is like an energy molecule that helps to burn fat, improve your cholesterol levels, raise energy,

---

Off the Grid with Diabetes

and improve your thyroid and pancreas function. It literally helps your heart and cells breathe.

As we age and our body begins to deteriorate (as the diabetic body does at a faster rate), the process of converting COQ10 into anti-oxidants begins to fail. Many researchers believe that COQ10 is a leading possible solution for late-stage heart disease patients, and even synthetic options are desirable. Naturally, you can find COQ10 in sardines, mackerel, beef heart and liver, lamb, pork, and eggs. You can also find COQ10 in spinach and broccoli.

You can supplement with artificial forms of COQ10, which may go by the name utiquinol. The best supplements will be in soft gel form and free of soy or gluten. 50 to 100 milligrams twice daily is a common dosage, but this is something you should verify with your doctor, because high amounts of this can cause your blood pressure to plummet.

Another heart supplement that is naturally occurring in the body is ribose, also known as D-ribose. Ribose is directly related to the production of other energy molecules that your body needs to keep your heart beating. Ribose is found throughout your body and provides an essential compound that forms part of our DNA. It's also a component of vitamin B2 and is widely used by athletes to help overcome muscle soreness. Ribose helps prevent heart failure by improving blood flow and carrying more oxygen to the heart. As a result, it can ease feelings of shortness of breath, fatigue, and other symptoms that are commonly associated with a heart condition. Ribose is therefore an excellent supplement for not only those with heart conditions, but also those who suffer from pain, soreness, stiffness, and chronic fatigue. You might even notice results within as little as twenty-four hours.

You'll find ribose in red meat, especially veal, but even then it's not in very high quantities. So, in order to supplement with ribose we're going to have to look at artificial supplements. Three to five grams daily is a common dosage, and you can find high-quality

---

What To Do If You Have Diabetes And All Hell Breaks Loose   **153** supplements in many stores. Be careful though, because ribose can lower your blood sugar dramatically, especially if you're already on blood sugar lowering drugs. Consult your physician first.

One of the best all around heart treatments is the hawthorn herb, which grows all over the world and looks a lot like mistletoe. Studies have proven that it can improve the symptoms of heart failure, fatigue, chest pain, and even an irregular heartbeat. Hawthorn is so effective because it increases the amount of blood your heart is pumping and even lowers blood pressure. Hawthorn also apparently protects against the free radicals that can do so much damage to your arteries. Hawthorn might be tough to get into your diet, unless you want to grow the herb yourself and eat the berries, leaves, and flowers. Otherwise, you're going to need to find an extract containing vitexin (the active ingredient in hawthorn). Take with caution and ease into it, because some people are sensitive and may experience dizziness, drowsiness, a drop in blood pressure, and even heart palpitations.

Another amino acid that many diabetics are deficient in is taurine, a building block for protein. Taurine also has antioxidant effects, so it helps to clear up free radicals that can hurt your brain, heart, pancreas, liver, and arteries. Taurine has been proven to help increase your body's sensitivity to insulin and get the sugar out of your system after you eat. Taurine can regulate your heartbeat, improve healing, regulate your blood pressure, protect the kidneys and liver, assist in the creation of pancreatic cells, and lower blood sugar. You will find taurine in lean meat, poultry, fish, and eggs. Vegans rarely get enough taurine, so they will need to supplement with 500 to 1000 milligrams daily.

Another supplement you can take, and one of my favorites, is resveratrol. It's the key ingredient in red wine that makes red wine a virtual health food. The problem, of course, is that wine contains a lot of sugar in the form of alcohol. Otherwise, resveratrol can improve cholesterol ratios, lower LDL, and is generally good

Off the Grid with Diabetes

for you. Resveratrol can inhibit the growth of cancer cells and generally shows great promise. But since we don't want to base a diet around drinking red wine, you should seek to find resveratrol in red or purple grapes, grape juice, organic nuts, and peanut butter. If these aren't an option for you, you might try 1000mg daily of polygonum cuspidatum, a Japanese knot wood shrub. The extract should be at least 50 percent resveratrol.

You're going to laugh at this next one, but seriously, I'm going to recommend chia seeds as one of the richest vegetarian sources of essential fatty acids. The fatty acids protect your brain, pancreas, blood vessels, and arteries, as well as your liver and heart. Chia seeds have been consumed by ancient societies, including the Aztecs and Mayans, and are one of the most nutrition-packed foods for their size. They're only the size of a flaxseed! Several athletes have been consuming these, and the mainstream media is picking up on them. They're also easy to consume because you don't have to grind them, and they have a longer shelf life.

Just one ounce of dried chia seeds contains nearly 5,000 mg of omega-3 fatty acids and 170 mg of calcium. Chia seeds absorb several times their weight in water, which helps you feel full and can therefore curb hunger and help you manage your weight. You may find that they help improve skin conditions, joint pain, and your immune function. You can buy organic chia seeds at health food stores and online, but make sure you only use the dark version of chia seeds, not white! Stick with the natural, proven dark chia seed and add it to just about any food in your diet.

While your heart is critical to your life and one of the most commonly affected organs, it is not the only organ that suffers. Many people, even those without diabetes, suffer from kidney failure and may not even know it. In fact, more than 25 million Americans have kidney disease. If you've had diabetes for ten years or more, the kidneys start to lose their effectiveness as the blood vessels that support the organs become diseased. Kidney

disease in diabetics is particularly bad and is a leading cause of a need for dialysis. Once your kidneys fail to this degree, your chances of living beyond three years fall rapidly. Because kidney disease is so dangerous and seems to so often go undiagnosed, let's review a few of the symptoms of kidney trouble now. Even if you don't have any of the symptoms, there may come a time when someone you know or love begins to manifest these signs, and a physician may not be available.

If you find there is a change in your urine—for example, if you suddenly need to urinate less often, or when you do urinate only a small amount of urine comes out—you should immediately go to the ER. If you feel a lot of pressure when you urinate, or if your urine is foamy or dark, like a strong tea, then you need to see a physician. If you see swelling in just one ankle and you've not injured yourself physically, then you might be suffering from an edema that is the result of your kidneys failing to properly remove fluid. Because this often manifests itself in only one of your legs, ankles, feet, or hands, this odd kind of swelling is often a sign of kidney failure.

Because your kidneys are responsible for the production of red blood cells, which help to deliver oxygen to the rest of your body, failure in the kidneys can lead to fewer red blood cells, anemia, and exhaustion. Sometimes these signs are misdiagnosed as chronic fatigue syndrome, fibromyalgia, and even depression. Anyone in this category who also suffers from high blood sugar should have their red blood cell count measured to make sure it's not a kidney-related problem.

Since your kidneys are responsible for removing waste from your bloodstream, if they're not working properly the waste will begin to build up, and one of the first signs is really itchy skin. I'm talking really severe itching, not the occasional itch we all get. Unfortunately, this kind of problem is also easily misdiagnosed, and you'll find yourself on an anti-histamine or steroid lotion when in reality it is your kidneys that are failing and

Off the Grid with Diabetes

causing this itching. If you develop this strange chronic itching and you think you are at risk for diabetes or already have it, it makes sense for a physician to check things out before you start treating other symptoms.

Another sign of kidney failure is really bad breath. This happens because the kidneys, not being able to filter your blood properly, miss a substance known as urea, and as it begins to build up you'll notice a strange, metallic taste in your mouth. Your food may even taste differently. If this happens, you have a sure sign of possible kidney deficiency. This same substance can cause you to feel nauseous, and you may feel like you're going to throw up. Even a tiny bit of food or soup can be impossible to keep down.

Another serious sign of chronic kidney disease is difficulty breathing because the fluid in your body starts to pool in your lungs. Since you may also be anemic, you don't have enough red blood cells carrying oxygen to your body, including your pulmonary capillaries where it is desperately needed. As a result you have shortness of breath or feel like you can't take a deep breath. Even a short duration of exertion will leave you feeling like you are drowning. Because of the symptoms, you are likely to be diagnosed as having a respiratory infection, pneumonia, or asthma. Obviously it is a serious condition, so make sure your physician considers the fluid buildup as a possible kidney issue.

Anemia can also lead to a problem in the brain, since it is starved for oxygen. You might have a problem concentrating or remembering things. I'm not talking about getting older and not being able to remember things at sixty like you did when you were twenty, but having trouble doing math or remembering what you did yesterday or the inability to finish a sentence. You might even get dizzy. These can all be connected to your brain being starved for oxygen.

Finally, if your kidneys themselves have fluid building up on them, cysts can form and pain will result. This lower back pain

 # Off the Grid with Diabetes

can also migrate down your leg, so it's easily thought to be arthritis or even sciatica! If you have this kind of problem, you may toss and turn all night trying to get comfortable.

Other than these signs, when your kidneys start to fail, there often isn't a pain that suddenly leads you to think, "Oh, my kidneys are failing." That's why if you have diabetes, high blood pressure, high cholesterol, hardening of your arteries, or a lot of chemical toxins in your body, you've got to be on guard for chronic kidney disease. While the medical world is focused on miracle cures to fix what we're doing to ourselves through diet and lifestyle, I want to share some changes you can make that will greatly reduce your chances of having kidney problems and may even help to restore lost kidney function.

Protein-rich foods have an adverse impact on your kidneys because your kidneys have a hard time sorting out the protein from the waste material. If you think your kidneys are already stressed, try to avoid the protein-rich foods and limit your intake to just a few times a week.

At the same time, fat can be problematic for the kidneys, because fat adds to the high levels of cholesterol in your blood, and as it builds up in your vessels, it puts a lot more pressure on your kidneys.

Salt is a problem too, because all that salt in your body causes you to retain water, which means your kidneys have even more fluid to filter out. It's not just the pinch of salt that you add to your foods that causes a problem; it's the sodium that is present in the processed foods we consume. Frozen dinners, processed meats, snack items like chips and popcorn, and prepared soups (like those terrible ramen soups) have huge amounts of sodium. All these are kidney killers.

Here are some ideas to improve kidney health and function. Use natural sea salt whenever possible, but generally look for additional flavor from peppers rather than salt. Salt substitutes

Off the Grid with Diabetes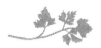

aren't a good idea because many of them rely on potassium, which, if it builds up in the blood, can cause other problems, just worsening the situation.

Avoid soda. Studies have shown that women who drink two cans of soda a day are nearly twice as likely to develop early kidney disease as those who don't drink soda. Soda is just terrible for you; it contains phosphorus, which isn't good for you in concentration, as well as high fructose corn syrup, which we talked about earlier. And, nearly half of all sodas containing high fructose corn syrup have been found to contain mercury in trace amounts! So, stick with water and low-fat and low-protein diet drinks, especially fruit and vegetable juices.

You should also look at supplementing with carnitine, an amino acid also known as L-carnitine. Your body manufactures this naturally, but if your kidneys aren't working properly, you may not have enough of it. Carnitine is also good for nerve regeneration, which helps to reduce pain. Carnitine can also combat high levels of free radicals and may also improve your insulin tolerance. You can find carnitine in lamb, dairy products, and wheat. Even better sources are fish, poultry, asparagus, avocados, and cashew butter. If you must use an artificial supplement, avoid D-carnitine because it is not the pure carnitine you need and isn't as easily absorbed by the body. 500 or 1000 milligrams three to four times a day with food is the normal dosage, but make sure you check with your doctor because some people are sensitive to carnitine.

An herbal supplement that I really like is horsetail or equisetum arvense, sometimes called shave grass or bottlebrush. The stems of this plant are a great source of silica, which helps to form collagen, a protein that is vital for health of ligaments, cartilage, and connective tissue. Silica is a great supplement and helps with pancreatic health, osteoporosis, and even hair and nail health. Horsetail also acts like a diuretic, helping to filter the blood and eliminate some of the fluid buildup that could be causing

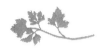

your kidneys a problem. You can get silica in whole grains, but rarely in high quantities, so you may need to look to an herbal supplement for this one. Try tinctures, teas, and all-natural, high-quality oral supplements.

B1 vitamin, also known as thiamine, helps to keep the nerves and brain healthy, and a deficiency in thiamine can lead to depression, nerve pain, muscle weakness, irritability, and muscle atrophy. A long-term deficiency can even lead to an enlarged heart, rapid heartbeat, and neurological problems. In lab tests, B1 has proven to have dramatic effects on the body's ability to reverse early-stage kidney disease among some diabetics. Thiamine is also known to have beneficial effects on the pancreas. You can get thiamine in whole grains, fortified cereals, meat, and yeast, but it's another example of something you may need a supplement to get. Look for thiamine pyrophosphate or a B-complex supplement with thiamine.

When your kidneys are losing the battle, one of the hormones that loses out is calcitrol, which is the end product of the absorption of vitamin D. There has long been a strong connection between vitamin D deficiency and Type 2 diabetes. Since vitamin D helps to lower blood sugar, protect the nerves, and improve insulin resistance and bone strength, there's not much downside to taking in some more vitamin D. Of course, the best source of vitamin D is the sun. Just fifteen minutes a day of sunbathing can get you all the vitamin D you need. However, we can't all sunbathe daily and as our bodies age, our ability to take vitamin D in through the skin decreases. If that's the case, you may want to look at a vitamin D supplement. High-quality vitamin D3 supplements may contain as much as 2,000 IU daily.

One way to combat anemia is pau d'arco bark, sometimes called taheebo or lapacho, an herb from the Amazon that appears to support red blood cell production and health. Experts think pau d'arco thins the blood and helps purify the kidneys of toxins. A

Off the Grid with Diabetes

natural source of pau d'arco is hydroquinone, the same substance that is used to treat sunspots. You can get this in over-the-counter form, or you can buy pau d'arco in extract, capsule, tablet, or liquid form. Pau d'arco is enjoyed by many people in tea form, which is how I would recommend you try it. Some of the side effects can be nausea or vomiting, and because it's a blood thinner, use caution if you are already on other blood thinners.

In China, a plant by the name of astragalus has long been used to boost immune function and treat heart and kidney disorders. It can even increase the effectiveness of some medications. It can help with high blood pressure and water retention. However, if you have Type 1 diabetes, you shouldn't take this unless your doctor recommends it.

Finally, I want to recommend a few herbal teas that can really help and that you don't have to worry about having an adverse interaction with any other medicine.

Chamomile is a popular tea that you have undoubtedly already heard of, and it's one of the best botanical treatments. In lab tests, chamomile not only helped to reduce blood sugar levels by 25 percent, it also helps to reduce muscle tension and produce an overall relaxation, similar to a mild sedative. This is why it is so popular!

I also want to recommend rooibos, which is also called African red bush tea. Rooibos contains polyphenols and minerals that help the pancreas, such as zinc, calcium, magnesium, manganese, iron, potassium, and copper. It is also a source of alpha hydroxy acid, something found in many skin-care products. Rooibos has been known to increase the strength of your capillaries as well, thanks to the presence of quercetin. When your capillaries improve, you will see an overall improvement in heart function, lower blood pressure, and better blood flow to your eyes, brain, kidneys, and your extremities.

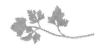

Bitter melon tea is derived from the fruit of the bitter melon and helps to lower blood sugar. This is great to drink after meals, especially if you indulge in some not-so-healthy foods. There are also bitter melon extracts sold as supplements, and these are much stronger than the tea, so if you really need a boost, you might want to consider the supplements. I find that after a meal, the tea is a great way to stabilize blood sugar and increase insulin secretion, which allows your muscles and fat to absorb the glucose and protect your kidneys.

If some of the effects of diabetes haven't been horrible enough thus far to persuade you to consider radical action, discussing neuropathy—the painful nerve damage that results from high blood sugar over a prolonged period of time—may get your attention.

Neuropathy can manifest itself in a variety of ways, from burning pain to faintness or dizziness when standing, loss of bladder control, balance problems, erectile dysfunction, poor coordination, muscle pain, numbness, shooting pain, tingling in the extremities, nausea and vomiting, the sensation of pins and needles, facial pain, and vaginal dryness.

Once you have neuropathy, treatment becomes a constant race to outrun the spread of nerve damage and get in front of the escalating pain. Of course, the medical profession has a lot of experience treating pain and can dial the dosage up higher and higher. But we want a natural approach that also offers hope for recovery. One of the best natural treatments is capsaicin, the compound that puts the hot in hot sauce. It works by numbing nerve endings and can help with arthritis in the fingers, elbows, and knees. It works even better than menthol-based treatments, which just mask pain with a cold sensation.

Capsaicin has worked for a lot of people who were in terrible pain that wasn't eased by other more traditional chemical treatments. Capsaicin works best when used in a preventive capacity, so rub it into the affected areas before you have an onset of pain. It will generate a burning sensation initially, but that will go away quickly and you'll find that your neuropathic episodes disappear! You can find all sorts of information about capsaicin on the web and in all the major drug stores.

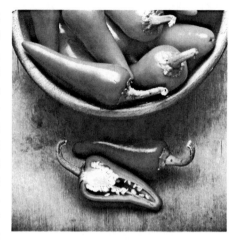

Some oral supplements that can help with neuropathy are alpha lipoic acid, curcumin, vitamin B12, the L-carnitine we discussed earlier. Alpha lipoic acid is a powerful antioxidant that can help to neutralize free radicals. It can also help other anti-C oxidants already in your body, like vitamins C and E and glutathione. Repeated studies over the years have shown that alpha lipoic acid helps to reduce pain and improve neuropathic symptoms.

Curcumin works by reducing blood sugar and pain sensitivity. Curcumin helps to counter the effects of nitric oxide, which can cause pain when it is produced in abundance. Because it's tough to ingest enough curcumin, you may need a supplement if you really want it to have an effect.

B12 has a great reputation and is a good all-around supplement. A deficiency of B12 can lead to a loss of the protective covering of your cells, increasing neuropathic pain. One of the best ways to get vitamin B12 is in methylcobalamin, which makes its way with the highest efficiency into the brain and nervous system, which is critical since that is the pain that we're dealing with here.

We already discussed acetyl L-carnitine, but in addition to helping your kidneys, it is also proven to be a great pain reliever. In fact, it has been sold in Europe as a prescription for nearly twenty years.

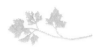 # Off the Grid with Diabetes

One additional way to help your body deal with neuropathy is finding the right balance of minerals in your life. As it concerns neuropathy, the really important minerals are calcium, magnesium, zinc, selenium, vanadium, chromium and copper. When you look to supplement with these minerals, make sure you get chelated minerals, which will penetrate your nerve tissue more easily. Synthetic brands are the ones sold in many common forms, so be sure to check. If you're eating spirulina, you may already be getting all the minerals you need and in the best possible form.

Nerve damage and loss of feeling in the feet is also a common experience for people with diabetes, especially those who have lived with undiagnosed diabetes for some time. One of the first signs of this problem is a sore or cut on the foot or leg that goes unnoticed until it becomes a blister or gets infected. If you have nerve damage in your body and you get even one ulcer, the odds of developing more ulcers and other complications are even greater, even if you are doing everything you can to combat the outbreaks.

Although anyone with diabetes can develop a foot ulcer, some people are more likely to get them. Native Americans are at the greatest risk, followed by African Americans and Hispanics. Additionally, the elderly and anyone who is on insulin are at a high risk of developing ulcers. But regardless of whether you are already in one of these high-risk categories, the following list will help you prepare and prevent the possibility of these terrible afflictions, which often result in amputation, something that would be particularly grave in an off-grid situation.

If you do some research online about the ways to prevent foot ulcers, you'll find lots of great suggestions, including wearing good shoes, checking daily for sores, and keeping the feet clean and dry. However, far and away the best answer is to reduce blood sugar! If we address the core issue rather than the side effects, we virtually guarantee we can prevent the ulcers and all but eliminate any risk of amputation!

Off the Grid with Diabetes

From your eyes to your toes, regulating and lowering your blood sugar minimizes all the dangers we want to avoid. Once we recognize that treating diabetes is no longer about treating the symptoms, the better off we will be. As with anything else, prevention is key. So, let's return to the list above—all good ideas.

When you get new shoes, you should invest in high-quality items, and break them in slowly. Don't wear them eight to twelve hours a day for a week, but for a few hours at a time, gradually increasing usage over a few weeks. When you take your shoes off, inspect your feet closely. You're looking for sores, cuts, splinters, ingrown toenails, and even cracked skin. Cracked heels are common in people with diabetes, and they can become a breeding ground for bacteria and fungus. Apply lotion daily to keep feet soft and moist, but otherwise you want to make sure your feet are cleaned vigorously and kept dry. One simple change is to make sure that you don't wear socks at night. Let those feet breathe whenever possible, but don't walk around barefoot! There is too much of an opportunity for injury. Avoid flip-flops and open toe sandals as well. If you've got corns, calluses, bunions, or other foot problems, see a podiatrist and get those addressed. There may come a time when a doctor isn't available.

One great preventive step is massage and reflexology, because this gets more blood moving in your limbs, bringing more oxygen to your feet. Any cardio exercise is great, but a foot massage in particular can help and it feels great too! However, you should be very careful with pedicures because of the risk of even the slightest injury and the risk of infection from improper sanitation between clients.

Unfortunately, no amount of preventive care can guarantee protection from an injury. For very small wounds, you can wash them with a salt-water solution, much like a contact lens or nasal irrigation solution you can find in many stores. You use saline rather than water because saline more closely resembles your body's natural fluids. Afterwards, apply a topical antimicrobial

Off the Grid with Diabetes

cream or ointment or triple antibiotic ointment to help speed healing and avoid infection.

An ulcer is a more serious wound and is beyond the scope of this chapter. However, anyone trained in biology may be capable of treating this kind of wound, even a veterinarian or dentist, who in an emergency can diagnose an infection and do basic surgery. But let's focus on what you can do to help your body fight off these challenges.

One of the most important supplements for your foot health is vitamin C. Vitamin C is necessary to make collagen, the substance that helps build strong bones and keep your skin soft and beautiful. The best sources of vitamin C are citrus fruits and green vegetables.

Of course, you can also supplement artificially with natural vitamins. Look for brands that contain bioflavonoids derived from fresh fruit. Try to avoid pharmaceuticals that drain your body of vitamin C, like aspirin, estrogen-containing drugs, diuretics, and anti-inflammatory drugs like ibuprofen.

Other great skin protectants are vitamin A and beta-carotene. They help to reduce lines in your skin and clean your tissues of free radicals. Foods that have a lot of beta-carotene include fruits and vegetables that are orange or red, such as carrots, yams, apricots, squash, pumpkin, cantaloupe, and mangoes. Other good sources are broccoli, collard greens, lettuce, kale, and spinach.

Vitamin E is also well known for its anti-aging effects on the skin and is found in a lot of moisturizers and skin care products. You can get vitamin E in walnuts, almonds, seeds, wheat germ, leafy greens, and egg yolks. Of course, you can also supplement, but make sure you only use natural forms of vitamin E. The synthetic versions aren't as well absorbed by your body.

Another familiar supplement we've mentioned is selenium, which works really well in conjunction with vitamin E. Not only

Off the Grid with Diabetes

is it a great free radical defense, protecting the skin, but it also boosts your thyroid protection, which helps prevent diabetes. It is even shown to reduce your risk for developing lung, colon, rectal, and prostate cancer. You can get selenium in Brazil nuts, seafood, meat, turkey, rice, and oatmeal, or supplement with selenocysteine or selenomethionate.

Another great skin protectant is zinc because it is critical to the manufacture of collagen. It can help improve your overall skin condition as well as helping to heal bedsores, ulcers, burns, wounds, and even common skin irritation. Zinc also contributes to thyroid hormone, like selenium, and may improve fat burning capabilities. You can find zinc in seafood (oysters and shellfish in particular), beef, and nuts. Lesser sources are dairy products, pumpkin seeds, and green vegetables. If you can't get these foods into your regular diet, a simple way to supplement is with zinc lozenges. Just one daily gives you a big boost of zinc.

Silica is an important supplement for us to consider, because it's found in every skin cell in your body. Silica also maintains your blood vessels, so it's great for people with heart disease. Silica can even help your hair and nails look more youthful. You'll find silica in beets, leafy vegetables, and brown rice, but you're not likely to get enough silica this way. The best way to supplement is with liquid silica orally. This helps your body absorb it more quickly, and you can even apply it directly to wounds, including hemorrhoids. If you find a supplement that contains both silica and horsetail, that is ideal.

There are also some over-the-counter aids that may be of use. Aveeno baths can help with irritations, rashes, eczema, insect bites, and poison ivy or oak. Calamine is the pink lotion that you've probably used at one time or another, maybe with chicken pox or poison ivy. It's a great skin protectant for sores, pain and itching, and Calamine Plus is a stronger version with numbing properties.

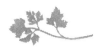

Off the Grid with Diabetes

Hydrocortisone comes in dozens of different forms and can be helpful for a wide variety of ailments. Domeboro is a powdered aluminum that you can mix with water and use as an astringent to help cool skin rashes, bug bites, athlete's foot, or poison ivy, oak, or sumac. However, you may find that these products aren't available in an emergency or off-grid survival situation. Some natural alternatives that are proven to mimic chemical solutions can be helpful. The saltwater saline solution is a good alternative to hydrogen peroxide, grapefruit seed oil could replace antifungal creams, and tea tree or tamanu oil can act as an antimicrobial ointment. Florasone, which is a natural non-steroid, is a great replacement for hydrocortisone, and aloe vera or shea butter is good for anti-itch situations, as is lavender essential oil.

In conclusion, dealing with all these diabetic symptoms begins with prevention. If you're borderline now, this is the time to take serious action, before you're in a critical, emergency off-grid situation. It's a lot easier to deal with these health problems while you have the full support of the medical community than when you may be fighting just for survival.

A good diet, lots of exercise, natural supplements and avoiding the really bad foods will accomplish most of what you need without the harmful side effects associated with the mass-produced chemical treatments, which may not be available down the road anyway.

However, because many of these solutions are found in nature, the most important thing to emphasize right now, as you have the time, is education. Becoming more familiar with the disease, how it progresses, and what those symptoms are will help you be prepared for any eventuality. Knowing how to respond to those symptoms will make you an invaluable member of your own family and any community that you are a part of. You may be able to save lives just with the simple application of a few basic treatments you've learned in this book.

Off the Grid with Diabetes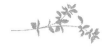

One of the important things to remember is to respond swiftly and aggressively to problems as they develop. A diabetic body is not like a healthy one that can be largely counted on to heal itself and fight off death. The diabetic body is already struggling just to live. It is seriously impaired and already fighting an all-out battle on numerous fronts, and it is doing so with weakened troops. Swift response to the symptoms and an aggressive treatment is critical. A simple toe injury, say, a nail that is poorly cut and becomes infected, can be life threatening to the diabetic in any situation, let alone one where a physician is unavailable and antibiotics are out of reach.

It's also important to remember that prayer should be a part of any treatment. I mention this last because it is the most important thing. You don't have to be a Bible-believing, church-attending person to believe in prayer; even atheist physicians recognize that prayer works!

Of course, the skeptics believe that the mindset of the suffering victim may be sufficient to generate miracles, which is an extraordinary claim since they can't prove how or replicate the result in the laboratory, but studies have repeatedly shown that people who are prayed for heal faster and more completely than those who are not prayed for, even when the person being prayed for doesn't know it or even rejects the whole idea! God is not bound by natural law, so don't leave Him out of your treatment plans. Pray without ceasing—before your injury, during treatment, and after recovery!

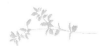

Off the Grid with Diabetes

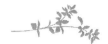

Chapter Nine:

What to Do Now

If you've reached the same conclusion that I have and the possibility of an off-grid lifestyle seems reasonable enough to warrant some preparation, you might find yourself overwhelmed with information and possibilities. It's easy to get overwhelmed with information, ideas, conflicting strategies, and what-if scenarios. I want to try to provide you with some reasonable advice to navigate this troublesome time. I have known people that got so overwhelmed that they simply threw up their hands in despair and said, "I'll just trust in God" and then made no efforts! That's not what God wants of us; He commanded Noah to build the ark, not wait around for floating debris to save him!

I believe the first step in any preparation should be evaluating, based on your location, what problems you are most likely to encounter. Making a list of scenarios based on where you live will help you make critical decisions for the future.

Let's begin with the most likely scenario— a natural disaster. What natural disasters have hit your area in the past? If you live in the far reaches of the north, you would be more susceptible to a blizzard. If you live in the Mississippi delta, a flood might be your primary threat. On the east coast it might be a hurricane. In the plains and mid-south it might be a tornado. In the West it could be an earthquake or drought.

Of course, these are just regular natural disasters. By what if something catastrophic was to happen? An earthquake measuring a 9 on the Richter scale would cause damage far beyond what a 7 or 8 would. Even if your house survives, you might find that all the water and gas lines are broken, electric lines are down, bridges are destroyed, and society has degenerated into looting and rioting. Preparing for just a normal earthquake won't suffice.

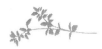 # Off the Grid with Diabetes

Similarly, if you live in the Mississippi delta, you have lived with floods your entire life. But what if you were to experience a once-in-a-millennia flood? Things would be very different. You might find that the sandbags you've always used to protect your property are easily washed away, and that instead of taking refuge in your home as an island, you're going to be on the roof looking for a helicopter that may never come. Or, what if you're safe in your home, like some of the refugees in New Orleans, but your community is cut off from civilization because of low-lying roads that are washed out and roving gangs are looting their way through the abandoned areas? Your normal level of preparation will not be sufficient for a life-changing catastrophe. Are you planning on drawing water from a nearby stream or river? What if a flood or hurricane has caused local sewers to overflow or malfunction and the water supply is now contaminated? You could have a year's worth of food in the basement, but if it's underwater or your house has been destroyed, it won't do you much good.

I believe you must strongly consider a survival plan with a relocation component. There are just too many things that can go wrong with your primary location that may make it uninhabitable. The sooner you consider this option and prepare yourself logistically (and emotionally, because walking away from your home and possessions can be very traumatic), the better off you'll be.

Probably the next most likely catastrophe to befall any community is an economic one. Looking at history and analyzing our own national problems, it's difficult to predict exactly what will happen and when, but it would reasonable to expect that hyperinflation is likely to be a part of our economic future. Preparing for a long, painful decline (not the overnight crisis some expect) seems most likely. How will you prepare if you lose your job or find your hours cut back dramatically? What if prices are going up every month at the rate they would normally increase in a year? The ATM may still work, there are no lines at the bank,

Off the Grid with Diabetes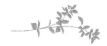

but you're gradually being suffocated. Even with income, you may find yourself in an extremely difficult situation. What if government rationing and price controls create two markets, like those that existed in the Soviet Union and still exist in Venezuela, North Korea, and Cuba today?

In this scenario, the food you are able to buy will be at a fixed price, but you won't be able to buy enough, so you will have to resort to the black market, where prices may be outrageous. Those who are dependent on welfare will see their safety net evaporate as those once-generous dollars no longer provide enough food. Even those with some wealth in the stock market, retirement accounts, or other liquid assets may suddenly find themselves poor, as those assets no longer purchase what they once did. As the generation that survived the depression recounts, the poor didn't realize there was a depression because they were already poor. But the middle class was destroyed, because the comforts and extras they were able to acquire to insulate them from market changes were gone or unaffordable. These economic changes will have exaggerated effects far beyond foreclosures as families are torn apart, crime rises, drug use escalates, and food shortages become the norm.

How will you survive in such an economic environment? It may be that there is no one to foreclose on your house, but what about feeding yourself or accessing health care? Unless you have stockpiled supplies, and better, know how to grow your own food and treat yourself, you're in trouble.

Another likely scenario in our future is a hostile health care environment, whether that is due to unaffordable coverage, rationing, long waits, shortage of medicines, or just selective health care. If tomorrow you were suddenly cut off from the health care system, if you couldn't go to a hospital, ER, your doctor's office, or the pharmacy, how would it impact your life? What if that situation persisted for a month? For six months?

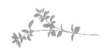# Off the Grid with Diabetes

If our country is the victim of another terrorist strike, as seems likely with the increasing hostility from Iran, how would your life be impacted? Unfortunately, the most likely and immediate impact is the increasing totalitarian environment we live in. Your movements might be restricted and certainly monitored. The medicines you buy and the quantities you may be authorized to keep could be limited.

If you've engaged in any activities that have put you on a watch list for domestic terrorism, such as blogging about constitutional issues, voting for tea party candidates, or speaking out against abortion or gay marriage, you might be considered a domestic terrorist and could be on the first lists for repression as the country begins to turn in on itself and persecute resisters. If you are confined to house arrest, for example, and not allowed to work or leave your home because of the threat you pose to domestic security, how will you provide for yourself and your family? How will you take care of your health?

And what of the more direct terrorist consequences? It's only a matter of time before a terrorist organization sneaks a backpack-sized nuke across the southern border and detonates it in a major city. New York and Washington have always been the top targets, but what if security measures there prevent the bad guys from executing their plans? Might they choose a second-tier city like Chicago, St. Louis, or Denver? What if they instead attack a nuclear power plant? Imagine the horror of a small nuclear device being detonated near a nuclear power plant. We know from the damage in Japan that a merely malfunctioning nuclear plant can cause problems thousands of miles away as radiation is released into the atmosphere, the food, and the water.

Also possible is an epidemic or plague that cannot be identified or brought under control. We've already had our brush with these possible diseases, like H1N1, which authorities have been able to "manage." But what happens when the strain is more

Off the Grid with Diabetes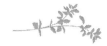

aggressive (i.e., it mutates faster than they can identify it and generate vaccines) or when the disease itself is more deadly— instead of just a flu, it causes the organs themselves to fail within days of infection. In such a situation, the worst case is that the government would quarantine the population to prevent the spread, which means that both the sick are denied treatment and healthy family members may be exposed (and of course denied treatment). Also, those who are not infected are denied access to normal care. A quarantine which lasted for a month or longer could see millions of otherwise healthy people die as they are left beyond the reach of basic medical care.

Having considered these possibilities and others that you have come up with on your own, it's time to personalize the situation. What are the medical needs you have that require ongoing care? What are likely medical conditions that you don't suffer from now that could be part of your future? What medical conditions do members of your immediate or extended family suffer from? What happens when these conditions go untreated for a significant period of time? What effect will extreme lifestyle changes have on these conditions? Many diseases are aggravated by stress, change in diet, and harsh conditions. Can you recognize the later stages of these conditions? Can you recognize the signs and treat them? Do you have offline, hard-copy information to help you treat these conditions so that when the Internet is no longer available you can diagnose and treat them?

Sometimes it is easy to feel overwhelmed by all the information. Therefore, I believe the prudent thing is to break your job into bite size pieces and tackle them one at a time. For example, let's assume that a three-day disaster is the most likely to occur, as would be expected from a bad blizzard, a tornado, a hurricane, or other short-term localized issue that will see the return to some sort of normalcy after just a few days. Things like this happen with relative frequency all over the world, and one need not be an end-times believer to accept that there could be a three-day

---

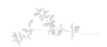

Off the Grid with Diabetes

disruption to our normal lives. What would our life be like if there was no fresh water for three days, or no electricity? What foods would spoil first? What unexpected problems would you have in your normal routine that you've not prepared for? Would cooking be more of a challenge than you thought? The only way to truly prepare for this kind of situation is to actually practice it by turning off the power and water for the weekend and doing a dry run. You will find all sorts of things that you didn't prepare for and didn't anticipate that will change your notion of what it means to be prepared.

The next scenario is a seven-day disruption, which is something that is relatively likely to happen during your lifetime. This requires thinking beyond just eating leftovers and eating whatever remains in your refrigerator. Your perishables will run out, and you'll be at the end of your first round of batteries. Water may become an issue if you've not adequately prepared or have a regular fresh water source. Fatigue and anxiety will be taking a toll at this point as your body struggles to adapt to a changed lifestyle and your mind is grappling with the possibility that this disruption might persist.

The next stage to consider is a thirty-day off-grid experience. It would take a real catastrophe to bring this about, and so the probability is less, but still possible. Water becomes the key issue, because it's not terribly difficult to store enough food for survival (although your diet is likely to be very different). Maintaining your health and sanitation are next after staying hydrated. Treating injuries quickly to avoid infection and protecting your property, food, and body from human or natural threats is key. Developing a routine that includes prayer, exercise, and some form of work is essential to a healthy survival attitude.

Once you begin to plan for a ninety-day routine, you are beginning to anticipate a true lifestyle off-grid. Ninety days is a sufficient enough disruption that life would look very different. Most of your prescriptions will likely have run out. Items you may have

Off the Grid with Diabetes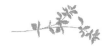

bought in bulk like toilet paper and diapers may have run out. Activities like washing your clothes are now taking up a fair amount of time and energy. Where do you get the fresh water for washing? How far do you have to walk? The energy you spend on this activity can be surprising. Some people who have survived physically may be starting to develop signs of mental illness as they struggle to adapt to the situation, realizing that life may never again be "normal." Or perhaps they are grieving for loved ones who have not survived. The mental and emotional strain will begin to set in as the realization that this new life is permanent can be a real burden.

Once you make it to six months, the changes in the population are dramatic. The young, old, sick, and injured who don't have a great support system will have died off. Even those who have stockpiled prescriptions will have run out. Those suffering from chronic diseases may begin to see those diseases take their natural course. By this stage, you need to be in the planning phase for long-term survival and can no longer just look to live on the foods you have stored away. You need to be gathering information about the outside world to see what is happening, whether you can expect there to be trade in food and other items, or whether you're going to be going at it alone.

Two seasons have passed by now, so you need to be evaluating your options for planting and raising crops, if you are not already. If you don't already have livestock, you need to be exploring options for acquiring some so you can round out your diet. No amount of stored food will last forever. You also need to be developing a trade, whether that is making things, hunting, repairing, or providing a service that has a value in the new economy. Hoarding things is not a good approach to maintaining life and security long term, and physical security will always be a problem if there is no law and order and anyone discovers that your survival mentality is one of storage rather than production.

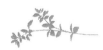# Off the Grid with Diabetes

By the time you get to one year, you're likely at the very limit of your stored food and supplies, unless you've been continually resupplying yourself. By now you should have developed a network of communication so you know what is going on in your local area and in the larger region. You should know whether it is safe to venture beyond your land into the local community, if physical security is an issue, if there are quasi-government organizations, and what the food supply situation looks like. Information is always a critical commodity, and it will be the same for you at this point as you begin to venture beyond the limits of what you have prepared for.

Review this list of different phases. Think through them step by step. How can you best prepare? Water should always be at the top of your list. You will not be able to store enough for your needs. You will have to have some renewable source of fresh water. Consider each stage and where your sources might be. Develop a backup source as well. What if you've had to abandon your primary residence and are at your plan-B location? You need to have sources of fresh water in each season. You can walk several miles to get a few gallons of water, but that's not practical in the long term. How will your access to water change with the weather or with a security threat? Are there other clusters of people who may be using that same water source?

After water, you need to have an immediate stockpile of any current, critical medications. Even if you are planning on making lifestyle changes, make sure you stockpile the medicines you're currently relying on so that you've got enough for ninety days minimum. Then, begin stockpiling over-the-counter treatment both for your chronic conditions and for minor injuries and other side effects of the off-grid lifestyle (like aspirin).

Next on the list would be medicines and treatments for potential conditions. Maybe you do not suffer from diabetes right now, but if your family members do (and they might end up with you) or

---

Off the Grid with Diabetes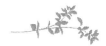

if you recognize some of the threats in your own lifestyle, you might want to consider stockpiling some of those medications. Of course, ideally you'll be looking for artificial and natural supplements to stockpile to treat these conditions as well, but a critical condition might best be treated with medication.

You also need to be considering the best long-term strategy for dealing with medical conditions—sustainable, homegrown foods and herbal treatments. This is last on your list, but it is the most important in the long term. I put it last because, since the crisis may come at any time, I want you to be able to put in your pantry today what you can get your hands on today, but the herbal survival garden that may save your life a year or two from now may take a season or two to get under way.

Of course all these things take time and money. You need to budget for both. I recommend that you develop an initial startup budget for the first round of supplies. This would be what you can afford out of pocket right now for the critical supplies as a starting point. You might find that $500 per person is a decent starting point. But this starting point is just that. The key to survival is the weekly or monthly contribution into your off-grid cache. You need to have a list you're working from every time you go to the grocery store, co-op, pharmacy, or herbal supply store of what you're buying and how it works into the rotation you've established.

At the same time, you should be scouting out the local sources of supplies wherever possible. It might be easy to go to Wal-Mart to stock up on supplies, but if a disaster hits your region, or even another region, Wal-Mart, relying on things from so far away, might be hit first by shortages. Having local sources for food, herbal supplies, and medicinal treatments is ideal to supplement your normal big-box suppliers.

The ideal scenario of course is to develop local, renewable sources for everything. What could be better than knowing the farmer who grows the corn or raises the goats or chickens? This is really

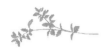

what you need to be working towards. We won't return to the dark ages just because the lights go off, but we will return to a nineteenth century lifestyle, and those who have the skills or relationships will be the ones who survive.

Another critical step on your journey should be a visit to the doctor. While you can, you need to go in for a full physical and get a complete-spectrum evaluation. You need all the results that you can print, evaluate, and save. You need to discuss your concerns with your doctor and share with him your proposed alternative treatments. Explain how you're preparing for a disaster and want to know how best to manage your medications in such a scenario. If you can get your doctor's personal contact information—not his office number—then you're a step ahead in a time of crisis. Have all your information printed on hard copy and available at your home for your family to access in event of an emergency.

You may also want to consider purchasing some information such as the **Physician Desk Reference** or publications like "When No Doctor is Available" that you can have on hand for dealing with off-grid medical treatments.

Once you have put these plans in motion, it's time to begin planning your own dietary and exercise changes so that if and when disaster strikes, you're in the best possible condition to face them. Begin implementing the green drink regimen, then a month later add the vitamin and supplements you've chosen, and then the following month begin phasing out the refined processed sugars, artificial flavorings, colors, and additives, the refined salt, and the white flour products. Remember not to do this all at once, because the shock to your body can be severe. Ease into it just like you're easing into your preparation regimen. But you must start! The more you delay, the likelier you are to put off indefinitely these important changes.

Off the Grid with Diabetes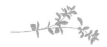

Next, you must begin living the off-grid lifestyle. It's not just a matter of storing a bunch of stuff in the corner of your garage or basement. It really is a lifestyle. Begin reading and informing yourself about how others are preparing. You don't have to agree with them on everything or adopt all their strategies, but you will undoubtedly learn from them.

You can also cautiously begin to network with other like-minded individuals in your community, people that you can approach if and when you are dealing with a crisis. Remember to always use caution and never brag about your own personal preparations. I can't overstate the importance of the practice sessions or dry runs. Practice one meal at a time, off grid. Then try a whole twenty-four hours with the electricity off. Then try a weekend. These experiences will be invaluable lessons.

Finally, don't forget to deal with the emotional and spiritual components. Make sure you've talked things through with your loved ones and friends. Have them read the same literature as you are so you can swap notes and contemplate your alternate future together. Discuss concerns and ideas. Develop a spiritual routine so you can enter a time of crisis and suffering with peace, confidence, and trust in God. The best material plans can easily be undone by a fractured family or a personal breakdown. Don't neglect this component—it could be the one that saves your life!

God bless you, and best wishes!

CPSIA information can be obtained at www.ICGtesting.com
Printed in the USA
LVOW130040151012

302751LV00003B/3/P